UNDERSTANDING ACCREDITATION IN LABORATORY MEDICINE

MANAGEMENT AND TECHNOLOGY IN LABORATORY MEDICINE

Series Editors: Gwyn McCreanor BSc, MSc, PhD, MRCPath
Roy A Sherwood BSc, MSc, DPhil
Guest Editor: John Sweetman BSc, MPhil, C Biol, MIBiol

UNDERSTANDING ACCREDITATION IN LABORATORY MEDICINE

DAVID BURNETT BSc, PhD
formerly Consultant Clinical Biochemist.
St Albans and Hemel Hempstead NHS Trust

A C B V E N T U R E P U B L I C A T I O N S

with generous support from:- Bayer plc - Diagnostics Division
Olympus Optical Co UK Ltd - Medical Products Division
Randox Laboratories Ltd
Roche Diagnostics

ACB VENTURE PUBLICATIONS
Chairman and Managing Editor - David Burnett.

MANAGEMENT AND TECHNOLOGY IN LABORATORY MEDICINE
Series Editors - Gwyn McCreanor and Roy A Sherwood

British Library Cataloguing in Publication Data.

A catalogue record for the book is available from the British Library.

ISBN 0 902429 20 5 ACB Venture Publications

Design and Illustration - Mike Webb of M J Webb Associates,
                          Helen Morrison of The Image Foundry Ltd.

Printed by Piggott Printers (Cambridge) Ltd.

Preface

The aim of this book is twofold, firstly, to introduce the subject of quality and accreditation systems in laboratory medicine using material from different systems, and secondly, to provide a source of practical information to assist laboratories preparing for accreditation. During the preparation it became clear that even in countries where English is the main language, definitions of every day laboratory terms, such as quality control, vary widely and therefore some care has gone into defining the terms used and to providing source references.

Where appropriate, material is used from the Pathology Laboratory of St Elsewhere's Hospital Trust. In this fictional laboratory, the pathologists work in complete harmony enabling the documentation to have a clarity of overall structure beyond belief. As this material has been prepared by the author from a vast array of material which was created by other humans, it is not necessarily the perfect solution to everyone's real life problems.

Not all quality and accreditation systems quoted in the book were designed for a pathology laboratory, but each system provides insights into what is considered appropriate for quality management in different settings. Sections of standards are quoted throughout the book, but the reader is advised to obtain the full text before embarking on implementation of any particular standard.

This book attempts a synthesis of experience in an important area of laboratory medicine but because no one individual can have practical experience with all quality and accreditation systems there will be errors and mistakes for which the author takes full responsibility. In the preparation of this book many colleagues throughout the world have listened patiently to my queries and provided valuable insights.

Thanks are due to members of my laboratory staff and in particular to my secretary, Rosemary Jones for struggling with my version of the English language, to Series Editors; Gwyn McCreanor of the Royal Free Hospital, London and Roy Sherwood of Kings College Hospital, London, and Guest Editor, John Sweetman of Corning Besselar Limited. Finally, thanks for the support of my family and friends who will be pleased to hear that the book is finally finished.

July 1996
David Burnett,

ACKNOWLEDGEMENTS

The Author thanks the following organisations and individuals for permission to reproduce or adapt material for certain figures in this publication. In case of some international standards, the limitations imposed on reproduction of more than a fixed percentage of the document makes it essential to obtain the complete standard for study. Full acknowledgement is made where appropriate in the text.

Permission to quote from standards and other material, (represented in the text in certain tables as shown in brackets):- British Standards Institution† (ISO 90001:1994), European Committee for Standardization† (EN 45001:1989), Organization for Economic Co-operation and Development†† (OECD), College of American Pathologists† (CAP-LAP), Clinical Pathology Accreditation (UK) Ltd† (CPA(UK)Ltd), National Council for Clinical Laboratory Standards† and the National Pathology Accreditation Advisory Council†.

Advisory, Conciliation and Arbitration Service UK†, Audit Commission UK†, BMJ Publishing Group London and Ross Anderson, Butterworth Heinemann Oxford, Churchill Livingstone Edinburgh, European Communities Confederation of Clinical Chemistry, Hewlett Packard Ltd, Kogan Paul London, Pan Books Ltd London, Medical Devices Agency† (Department of Health UK), Office Official Publications of the European Communities,† Royal College of Pathologists UK†

Excerpts from the Health and Safety Executive† documents are Crown Copyright and are reproduced with the permission of the Controller of HMSO.

---

†indicates that the full address is given in Appendix 1.

Contents

Chapter 1

What is accreditation?

INTRODUCTION

Before giving an account of the characteristics, elements and history of accreditation systems it is necessary to look at the usage of the word *'accreditation'*, and in particular to examine its meaning in contrast to the term *'certification'*.

In common usage* to *accredit* means 'to certify or guarantee someone or something as meeting required standards', and to *certify* means to endorse or guarantee that certain required standards have been met. This means that accreditation and certification in common usage have a similar meaning. However, the International Organisation for Standardisation (ISO) in ISO/IEC Guide 2 'General terms and their definitions concerning standardisation and related activity' draws a distinction between the two words. The definitions are given in Figure 1.1.

Accreditation

Procedure by which an authoritative body gives formal recognition that a body or person is competent to carry out specific tasks.

Certification

Procedure by which a third party gives written assurance that a product, process or service conforms to specific requirements.

ISO/IEC Guide 2 General terms and their definitions
concerning standardisation and related activity

Figure 1.1   Definition of accreditation and certification

It will be apparent as we examine different quality and accreditation systems, that in systems which are more commonly called *accreditation systems* whether an organisation meets certain standards is decided by peer review (an authoritative body), whereas in a *certification system* it is an independent third party, sometimes with specialist input, that guarantees adherence to standards.

---

*The Collins English Dictionary 3rd Edition updated 1994   ISBN 0 00 470678-1

In healthcare, the term accreditation is commonly used in three distinct ways which are shown in Figure 1.2.

Accreditation can recognise.....

- the fitness of a person to carry out a particular task.

- a health care facility or post in that facility as suitable for training purposes.

- a health care facility as having reached the standard required to carry out a prescribed function.

Figure 1.2   Usage of the term 'accreditation'

In this book the last usage will be assumed unless a specific reference is made to the contrary. However, the different ways in which the word accreditation can be used must be remembered when considering what a particular accreditation system may or may not encompass. This chapter will start by examining:

- the characteristics of accreditation systems.

- the elements of an accreditation system.

- the history of hospital and laboratory accreditation.

and conclude by outlining the distinctive ways in which accreditation of hospitals and laboratories may be sought.

CHARACTERISTICS OF ACCREDITATION

The words in italics in the definition given in Figure 1.3 bring out the main characteristics of accreditation systems. In the early development of accreditation systems, professionals come together *voluntarily* to formulate a set of *standards* that are seen as representing current views on good practice. An important part of the activity is seen as educational, and facilities (laboratories) *voluntarily* agree to be assessed or *measured* against the standards.

'Professional and national *recognition* reserved for facilities that provide *quality* healthcare. This means that the particular healthcare facility has *voluntarily* sought to be *measured* against high professional *standards* and is in *substantial compliance* with them'

Anon

Figure 1.3   A definition of accreditation in health care

If the facility is seen to be in *substantial compliance* with the standards, then within the professional framework appropriate *recognition* is given.

In countries where the conduct of clinical pathology becomes increasingly subject to legislation, some of these features may be in danger of being lost in over-regulation. In particular the voluntary and educational aspects can too easily be displaced by the emphasis on inspection and compliance. However, governments will often recognise the originating organisations as accrediting or certifying agencies, thus preserving the valuable contribution that such agencies make to improving standards.

ELEMENTS OF AN ACCREDITATION SYSTEM

There are three basic elements of an accreditation system. The first element is an accreditation board, typically the membership consists of representatives of professional bodies and health care organisations together with government observers. In some countries such as the Netherlands, the consumer interests are directly represented This is clearly important for the credibility of the accreditation process and obviates the criticism which is sometimes made, i.e. that professionals organise accreditation for their own self-interest. It is this body that confers accreditation and is responsible for the conduct of the organisation.

The second element is the set of standards and their supporting documentation. They are generally written to reflect and represent best practice and are kept under review by expert practitioners in the area. Further discussion on standards will be found in the next chapter.

Finally, there are the inspectors, surveyors or assessors who are chosen and trained to certify compliance with the standards. This is done by scrutiny of submitted applications followed by inspection visits. A laboratory can fail, or be given full or conditional accreditation. In the case of conditional accreditation, recommendations for improvements are made and a time for demonstrating compliance is specified. Additionally, there is a formal mechanism of appeal in the event of a laboratory being in disagreement with the recommendations following the inspection visit.

These elements may be more difficult to tease out in countries such as the USA, Canada and Australia, which have a federal structure, complex legislation and where significant autonomy is retained by the constituent states or provinces. Where regulatory and licensing activity has developed, the granting of accreditation may be blurred with licensing or with being recognised for receipt of payment from government or privately funded health care insurance schemes.

APPROACHES TO ACCREDITATION

There are a number of distinct ways in which clinical pathology laboratories can seek recognition 'as having reached the standard required to carry out a prescribed function'. The route that is followed in a particular country is in part determined by historical antecedents in that country or by the prescribed function of the laboratory. In countries such as the USA, Canada and Australia in which hospital accreditation has a significant history, the *laboratory accreditation* systems developed for clinical pathology laboratories tend to encompass both preanalytical and postanalytical phases of the testing process as well as the analytical aspects of a laboratory. They require definition of the head of department, participation in external quality assessment schemes and a relationship to the consumers of the service, the patients or their clinicians.

If a laboratory wishes to be recognised for purposes of testing chemicals to obtain data on their properties and/or their safety with respect to human health or the environment, then it will seek to be in compliance with the principles of *Good Laboratory Practice* (GLP). In this context the word 'principles' has much the same meaning as 'standards' (see Chapter 2). GLP is concerned with a narrower range of activities than the laboratory accreditation schemes described above. It is limited to the organisational process and conditions under which laboratory studies are planned, performed, monitored, recorded and reported. Nevertheless, the experience gained by practitioners of GLP has contributed greatly to the development of laboratory accreditation. Although GLP is formally intended for pre-clinical studies, some codes of Good Clinical Practice (GCP) such as the World Health Organisation (WHO) Guidelines for Good Laboratory Practice (1994) for trials on pharmaceutical products, specify in paragraph 4.7 that 'The trial site must have adequate facilities, including laboratories, equipment and sufficient medical, paramedical and clerical staff to support the trial. All laboratory assays must be validated and principles of Good Laboratory Practice (GLP) should be observed'.

Accreditation schemes are now being developed which are based on *International Standards* such as the ISO 9000 series of quality standards published by the International Organisation for Standardisation (ISO) and the EN 45000 series of standards prepared under the mandate of the Commission of European Communities (ECC) and the European Free Trade Association (EFTA) by the joint European Standards Institution's (CEN/CENLAC) Committee Group on Certification. At first sight, the terminology of the ISO 9000 series of standards may be unfamiliar to the laboratory professional, and the EN 45000 standards appear to focus on the analytical aspects of laboratory function, and do not seem applicable to a clinical pathology laboratory. However, thoughtful interpretation of these standards is bringing together some of the best aspects of the other approaches and making a new and valuable contribution to the history of laboratory accreditation.

The initial impetus for establishing hospital or laboratory accreditation schemes normally comes from health care professionals themselves motivated, at best by a concern for standards of patient care, or at least by enlightened self interest. After this first phase, during which government agencies sometimes provide financial support or seek observer status, there inevitably follows some regulatory activity. Political expediency seems to determine the speed with which governments act, and is generally in response to some level of public concern or to a desire to regulate public expenditure on health care.

HOSPITAL ACCREDITATION

In 1912, at the Third Clinical Congress of Surgeons of North America, a proposal was made which led to the formation of the American College of Surgeons in the following year. At the same congress a resolution was put forward which required, 'that some system of standardisation of hospital equipment and hospital work should be developed, to the end that those institutions having the highest ideals may have proper recognition before the profession, and that those of inferior equipment and standards should be stimulated to raise the level of their work. In this way patients will receive the best type of treatment, and the public will have some means of recognising those institutions devoted to the highest ideals of medicine'.

In 1917 the College established a hospital standardisation programme and over the next two years surveyed 692 hospitals of a hundred beds or more. Only eighty-nine hospitals surveyed met the standards and some of the most prestigious hospitals in the country failed to meet the most basic standards. As a result of this work *The Minimum Standard* was published in 1919. This quite remarkable document contains, amongst other important features, Section 5 which details the specific requirement for diagnostic and therapeutic facilities (Figure 1.4).

That diagnostic and therapeutic facilities under competent supervision be available for the study, diagnosis, and treatment of patients, these to include, at least:-

(a) a clinical laboratory providing chemical, bacteriological, serological, and pathological services;

(b) an X-ray department providing radiographic and fluoroscopic services.

Figure 1.4   Section 5 of The Minimum Standard

Dr Franklin Martin one of the individuals who developed the content of *The Minimum Standard*, said in 1934 that it was intended to 'safeguard the care of every patient within the hospital by insisting upon competence on the part of the the doctors, and upon adequate clinical and pathological facilities to insure correct diagnosis; by a thorough study and diagnosis in writing for each case; by a monthly audit of the medical and surgical work conducted in the hospital during the preceding interval; and by prohibiting the practice of division of fees under any guise whatsoever'.

By 1950, the College had approved over half the hospitals in the USA, but the increasing sophistication of medical care and the growing number and complexity of modern hospitals, combined with the emergence of non-surgical specialities after World War II, required that the standards be revised and the scope of the survey expanded. After lengthy discussion the American College of Physicians, the American Hospitals Organisation, the American Medical Association and the Canadian Medical Association, joined the American College of Surgeons to form the Joint Commission on Accreditation of Hospitals (JCAH), as an independent non-profit making organisation.

In 1959, the Canadian Medical Association withdrew to participate in the formation of the Canadian Council for Hospital Accreditation (CCHA). Hospital Accreditation in Canada is now administered by the Canadian Council on Health Facilities Accreditation.

Some fifteen years later, in 1974, the Australian Council on Healthcare Standards (ACHS) was established by the Australian Medical Association (AMA) and the Australian Hospital Association (AHA), its main objective being 'to facilitate, in co-operation with healthcare professionals, the development of an optimum level of care in hospitals and healthcare institutions throughout Australia'. In 1981 the Catalonian province of Spain implemented the first hospital accreditation programme in Europe.

In the United Kingdom, moves towards hospital accreditation were initiated by the Quality Improvement Programme of the King's Fund Centre. Following discussions with senior health professionals and representatives of professional bodies towards the end of 1988, a pilot project was established early the following year. Its aims were threefold:

- to develop a comprehensive framework of organisational standards for an acute hospital which could be applied nationally.

- to look at the process of assessing a hospital's progress towards meeting those standards.

- to assess the level of acceptance for a national programme of organisational audit.

After reviewing models of organisational accreditation from the USA, Canada and Australia, a system based on the Australian standards was adapted for the UK. The Organisational Audit programme between 1990 and 1995 has worked with two hundred acute National Health Service hospitals and independent hospitals throughout the UK. There is now a demand for the audit to be coupled with the granting of accreditation.

LABORATORY ACCREDITATION

In the United States of America the first scheme specifically designed for clinical laboratories was the Laboratory Accreditation Programme (LAP) initiated by the College of American Pathologists (CAP) in 1961. Its primary goal is that of laboratory improvement through voluntary participation, professional peer review, education, and compliance with established performance standards. The programme examines all aspects of quality control and quality assurance in the laboratory, including test methodologies, reagents, control media, equipment, specimen handling, procedure manuals, test reporting, and internal and external proficiency testing and monitoring, as well as personnel safety and overall management practices.

The programme is recognised by the Joint Commission on Accreditation of Healthcare Organisations (JCAHO), and CAP accredited laboratories are not surveyed by a Joint Commission surveyor. However, a physician surveyor will review information on intra-departmental requirements on safety and monitoring and evaluations of the quality and appropriateness of patient care. The programme is also recognised to have a deeming authority under the Clinical Laboratory Improvement Amendments of 1988 (CLIA'88) and accreditation by CAP is accepted in lieu of federal inspection by the Health Care Financing Administration (HCFA).

In Canada, laboratory accreditation remains the responsibility of the different provinces and as yet no federal approach has been developed. In 1971 in the province of British Columbia, a Diagnostic Accreditation Programme (DAP) was established under the joint sponsorship of the College of Physicians and Surgeons of British Columbia and the British Columbia Medical Association in response to governmental changes to the existing Medical Services Act Regulations. These changes created a licensing system for diagnostic laboratories and directed the referring physician to send patients to public in preference to private facilities. The DAP has six subcommittees, one of which relates to clinical laboratories excluding anatomic pathology which has a separate subcommittee. The clinical laboratories subcommittee carries out its mandate in three distinct ways:

- by regular on-site inspections of laboratory facilities
- by mandating and monitoring external proficiency programmes
- by designating and defining guidelines and standards for laboratory practices.

Laboratory accreditation in Australia started in the late 1960's with approaches by professional bodies to the Government, motivated by concern that certain services were of an unacceptable standard. Reaction from government was slow, but in 1979 the National

Pathology Accreditation Advisory Council (NPAAC) was established, its role being to act as a co-ordinating and standard setting body, with inspection and accreditation being the responsibility of State and Territory governments. Following the formation of NPAAC, only limited progress was made to introduce necessary State or Commonwealth legislation. Only after a number of reports that included the Parliamentary Public Accounts Committee's report on fraud and over-servicing in pathology, did government respond by creating the legal basis for a national Commonwealth scheme, the Health Legislation Amendment Act (1986).

Three levels of organisation in the laboratory accreditation process can now be recognised:

- the national standards setting body (NPAAC)
- the accrediting agencies prescribed in State or Commonwealth legislation
- the inspection agencies.

The National Association of Testing Authorities (NATA), because of its early practical experience with the Royal College of Pathologists of Australasia, is recognised as the principal inspection agency. Interestingly, the Commonwealth has accepted the Royal Australian College of General Practitioners (RACGP) as an approved inspection agency in Victoria with respect to services provided by medical practitioners to their patients.

In the United Kingdom in 1988, an *ad hoc* committee of The Royal College of Pathologists (RCPath) was formed to explore the feasibility and desirability of establishing a laboratory accreditation scheme. After an initial pilot study, a steering committee was formed with representatives from the College, the Association of Clinical Pathologists, the Association of Clinical Biochemists, the Institute of Medical Laboratory Sciences, the Institute of Health Service Managers and the Independent Health Care Association, together with observers from government health departments, the Advisory Committee on the Assessment of Laboratory Standards and the King's Fund.

Following a project development programme spanning three years, Clinical Pathology Accreditation (UK) Ltd. (CPA), was incorporated on the 6th January 1992. This non-profit making enterprise is owned by the share holders represented on the original steering committee. The main documentation consists of an application form and handbook. Forty-four standards were adopted, forty-one of which are common to all disciplines in pathology. These standards owe much to the laboratory sections of accreditation documents used by the Canadian Council on Health Facilities Accreditation, the Australian Council on Healthcare Standards and the King's Fund, London.

GOOD LABORATORY PRACTICE

The principles of 'good laboratory practice' have for many years been implemented voluntarily by laboratories in the private and public sector. However, in the early 1970's systematised governments began to look at good laboratory practice as a means to control laboratory activities. In 1973 the New Zealand Government enacted the Testing Laboratory Registration Act, which defined 'the testing laboratory' to include staff records, procedures, equipment and facilities. The Act established a testing laboratory registration council whose job it was 'to promote the development and maintenance of good laboratory practice in testing'. The significance of this legislation, and that promulgated in the same year in Denmark, was to give private and public laboratories something with which they could confirm their credibility or the quality of their research.

In July 1975, at a hearing of the subcommittee of health of the Senate Judiciary Committee, certain employees of the Food and Drug Administration (FDA) made allegations of improprieties on the part of Searle Laboratories in conducting and reporting animal safety standards through food and drug administration in the USA. Searle agreed to co-operate fully with the FDA in a thorough investigation of their pre-clinical research. At the same time, Hasleton Laboratories (USA), a contract laboratory used by Searle, was also investigated. As a result of these investigations, scientists at Searle produced a document entitled 'Good Laboratory Practice' (GLP) which was submitted to the FDA and the Pharmaceutical Manufacturers Association (PMA) in January 1976.

In August of the same year the FDA released draft principles of GLP based very much on the original Searle document and instigated an inspection programme. The final GLP regulations were published in the Federal register on 22nd December 1978 and became a legal entity in the United States on 20th June 1979. Revised regulations were published on the 4th September 1987 in the Federal Register entitled 'Good Laboratory Practice Regulations, The Final Rule'. Under these regulations inspections are carried out approximately every two years by the FDA, who also reserve the right to inspect any foreign laboratory that submits data to it.

In 1979 the Organisation for Economic Co-operation and Development (OECD)*, of which the USA is a member, started work to develop international principles of GLP. In 1982 the OECD published 'GLP in the testing of chemicals - Final Report of the OECD Expert Group on Good Laboratory Practice'. Various European Community (EC)

---

* The OECD, formed in 1961, is an instrument for international co-operation among industrialised member countries on economic and social policies. Countries include Australia, Austria, Belgium*, Canada, Denmark*, Finland, France*, Germany*, Greece*, Iceland, Ireland*, Italy*, Japan, Luxembourg*, Mexico, The Netherlands*, New Zealand, Norway, Portugal*, Spain*, Sweden, Switzerland, Turkey, United Kingdom*, United States of America. Countries marked * are also EEC member states.

Directives and Proposals between 1979 and 1988 indicated that OECD GLP standards should be used when carrying out safety tests on various specific types of chemicals including human and veterinary medicines, and embraced the concept of mutual acceptability of test data. Several countries including the UK, Holland, USA and Japan have governmental inspection groups.

INTERNATIONAL STANDARDS

There are two distinct systems that now have a relationship to the activities of the International Organisation for Standardisation, the ISO 9000 series of Quality System Standards and the European EN 45000 series of standards for testing laboratories.

ISO 9000 QUALITY SYSTEM STANDARDS

The development of Quality System standards will have different origins in different countries but a brief history of such standards in the United Kingdom is important because it is very significant in the development of the ISO 9000 standards. In the United Kingdom the origins of the British Standards Institution (BSI) which publishes British Standards (BS) can be traced back to the British Engineering Standards Committee set up in 1901. This subsequently became the British Engineering Standards Association in 1918 and received a Royal Charter in 1929, finally being renamed the British Standards Institution in 1931 to recognise an increasing involvement outside engineering. The BS 5750:1987 Quality System Standards were largely based on Defence Standard 5 which was drawn up by the Ministry of Defence (UK) influenced by the US military and NATO and used for defence supplies procurement.

In 1987 a number of countries ratified an agreement recognising an International Quality System Standard, the ISO 9000:1987 series. These are the direct equivalents of BS 5750:1987 and are widely recognised throughout the world. The International Organisation for Standardisation was formed in 1946 and ISO members are the national standards bodies of the different participating countries. As of 31st December 1991, it had 72 member bodies, 18 correspondent members and organised 174 technical committees, 630 subcommittees and 1827 working groups.

In 1994 the ISO 9000 series of standards were revised by ISO/TC 176 the 'Quality management and quality assurance' technical committee (TC) of the International Organisation for Standardisation, and adopted by ISO and the European Committee for Standardisation (CEN) following a parallel voting procedure. Published in Europe as the EN ISO 9000:1994 series, these standards replace the EN 29000:1987 series and in accordance with the Common CEN/CENELEC Rules the following countries have to implement these European standards: Austria, Belgium, Denmark, France, Germany, Greece, Iceland, Ireland, Italy, Luxembourg, Netherlands, Norway, Portugal, Spain, Sweden, Switzerland, and the United Kingdom. Although not specifically relating to laboratories, the ISO 9000:1994 series of Quality Systems Standards are important standards which are embraced increasingly by organisations requiring to show that their products meet stated quality standards. The range of these standards is described further in the next chapter.

EN 45000 STANDARDS

In addition to the development of the ISO 9000 series described above, of most importance to laboratory accreditation are the ISO/IEC Guides (see Figure 1.5). These guides are published jointly with the International Electrochemical Commission (IEC), an older body started in 1906.

ISO/IEC Guide 2: 1991	General terms and their definitions concerning standardisation and related activities
ISO/IEC Guide 25:1990	General requirements for the competence of calibration and testing laboratories
ISO/IEC Guide 43:1984	Development and operation of laboratory proficiency testing
ISO/IEC Guide 58:1993	Calibration and testing laboratory accreditation systems-General requirements for operation and recognition

Figure 1.5   The ISO/IEC Guides

The International Laboratory Accreditation Conference (ILAC), which is an informal organisation started in 1977, has been the driving force behind the ISO/IEC Guide 25 'General requirements for the competence of calibration and testing laboratories'. In the European Union (EU), the EN 45000 series of standards have been developed, of which the first EN 45001 'General criteria for the operation of testing laboratories' was based upon the ISO/IEC Guide 25. The standards are prepared under the mandate of the Commission of European Communities (ECC) and the European Free Trade Association (EFTA) by the CEN/CENELEC Committee Group on Certification. These standards are considered by a number of European countries to be too narrow in scope to encompass the work of a pathology laboratory, as distinct from a testing laboratory. In particular, there is no requirement for the professional standing of the Head of Department, nor is there a requirement to participate in external quality assessment schemes or to make appropriate use of results from such schemes. In Europe there are a number of initiatives at present to adopt a form of ISO/IEC Guide 25/EN 45001, which is more appropriate to pathology laboratories.

FURTHER READING

Batjer J D. The College of American Pathologists laboratory accreditation programme. Clin Lab Haematol 1990; **12** (Suppl 1):135-138

Brooks T. Standards and Accreditation. King's Fund News 1989; **12**:2-3

Burnett D. Laboratory Accreditation: an overview. JIFCC 1993, **5**:146-151

Hynes A F, Lea A R, Hailey D M. Pathology Laboratory Accreditation in Australia. Aust J Med Lab Sci 1989; **10**:12-16.

Pathology department accreditation in the United Kingdom: a synopsis. J Clin Pathol 1991; **44**:798-802

Roberts J S, Coale J G, Redman R. A history of the Joint Commission on Accreditation of Hospitals. JAMA 1987; **258**:936-940

White G H. Accreditation: The Australian Experience. Ann Clin Biochein 1996; **33**:273-283

World Health Organisation Guidelines for Good Clinical Practice, Geneva, 1994.

Chapter 2

Standards, guidelines, criteria or principles?

WHAT IS A STANDARD?

No quality or accreditation system can be successfully organised without a great deal of thought being given to the standards upon which such a system is dependent. In the introduction to EN 45020:1993 (Glossary of terms for Standardization and related activities) the use of the English word *standard* in science and technology is described as having two different meanings, the first as a 'normative document' and the second as a 'measurement standard'. Normative in this context means 'implying, creating or prescribing a norm or standard'. In this book the word is used in its first sense and not in its narrower sense of being a measure or reference against which a method or instrument can be calibrated. The definition of a standard as a normative document is given in Figure 2.1. The footnote to this definition says that standards should be based on the consolidated results of science, technology and experience and aimed at the promotion of optimum community benefits. The use of the word standard as a normative document applies in the case of the international standards ISO 9001:1994 and EN45001:1989.

'A Document, established by consensus and approved by a recognised body, that provides, for common and repeated use, rules, guidelines or characteristics for activities or their results, aimed at the achievement of the optimum degree of order in a given context'

EN 45020:1993 Glossary of terms for Standardization and related activities.

Figure 2.1   A standard as a normative document

However the word 'standard' and its equivalents in contemporary English usage is used in a different way in other accreditation systems. Figure 2.2 lists a number of words that are used in a similar way to the word standard and it is useful to examine their meaning in definitions taken from a dictionary of contemporary usage of the English language. It can be seen by reference to Figure 2.2 that the terms 'guideline', 'criterion', and 'principle' are all defined by reference to the word 'standard'. Schemes such as the OECD Principles of Good Laboratory Practice, the College of American Pathologists-Laboratory Accreditation Programme and Clinical Pathology Accreditation (UK) Ltd system use the word standard or its equivalents in this contemporary sense.

Standard	'an accepted or approved example of something against which others are judged'. 'a level of excellence or quality'.
Guideline	'a principle put forward to set **standards** or determine a course of action'
Criterion	'a **standard** by which something can be judged or decided'.
Principle	'a **standard** or rule of conduct'

Figure 2.2   Standard, guideline, criterion, and principle

DEFINITION OF QUALITY

Having defined a standard as 'a level of excellence or quality', we must attempt a definition of quality before turning to its assessment or to measuring compliance with standards which purport to represent quality.

The internationally approved definition of quality (ISO 8402:1994, Quality management and quality assurance-Vocabulary) is given in the first section of Figure 2.3. The term entity is defined as 'item that can be individually described and considered'. The stated or implied needs are translated into 'requirements for quality' which are considered to be 'an expression of the needs or their translation into a set of quantitatively and qualitatively stated requirements for the whole characteristics of an entity to enable realisation and examination'. Additionally the 'requirements of society' must be taken into account in terms of any 'obligations resulting from laws, regulations, rules, codes, statutes and other considerations'.

'The totality of characteristics of an entity that bear upon its ability to satisfy stated or implied needs'

ISO 8402:1994 Quality management and quality assurance -Vocabulary

'A blood glucose result measured on the correct specimen, that is accurate, timely and properly interpreted is a quality product or service'

Anon 1995

Figure 2.3   Definitions of quality

The earlier version of ISO 8402 published in 1986 defined quality as 'the totality of features and characteristics of a product or service that bear upon its ability to satisfy stated or implied needs'. The introduction of the term entity into the newer definition of quality is not favoured by the British Standards Institution (BSI) who say in the national forward to BS EN ISO 8402:1995 (which is identical to ISO 8402:1994), "the principal concern is the use of the term 'entity' throughout the standard. In this respect, users may prefer to adopt the convention of EN 45020:1993, General terms and their definition concerning standardisation and related activity which considers the proper subject of standardisation to be 'product or service' not 'entity'. The term 'entity', in its all embracing sense, can give rise to ambiguity in definitions, for example, when applied to a 'person' or 'body'".

To move back to firmer ground, in the British Standard (BS 4778: Part 2 1991) a quality vocabulary of national terms, there is a useful discussion of the concept of quality. In summary, it says that the word 'quality' is often used for several distinct purposes, firstly in a 'comparative sense' or 'degree of excellence' whereby products or services are ranked on a relative basis; secondly in a 'quantitative sense' used in technical evaluations; and finally and most useful for laboratory medicine as 'fitness for purpose' which relates the evaluation of a product or service to its ability to satisfy a given need. This final definition is given life in the second part of Figure 2.3 in a form that will be readily understood by all those working in laboratory medicine and is a clear expression of the 'requirements for quality'.

STRUCTURE, PROCESS AND OUTCOME

Donabedian in 1966 proposed three questions which could be asked about the quality of an episode of health care; what facilities were used?, what was done?, and what was the result for the patient? The terms he used of structure, process and patient health outcome (usually and misleadingly abbreviated to outcome) are the three components of quality that Donabedian (1980) described as being capable of assessment or evaluation. (Figure 2.4).

Structure

The availability and organisation of resources (staff, buildings, equipment, consumables etc.) required for the delivery of a product or service

Process

The delivery of a product or service (analysis including internal quality control, reporting, interpretation, consultation and external quality assessment)

(Patient Health) Outcome

The alteration in the health status of an individual (clinical audit)

Figure 2.4   A Framework for quality assurance

In describing quality assessment in the context of health care, he regarded the *process* of care as the primary object of assessment. Process, in the laboratory context, would include all operational activities associated with the collection, transport, reception and registration of specimens or samples, their analysis and reporting. Aspects of accreditation associated with process are discussed in Chapters 9-10 and many of these can be assessed, such as turnaround time for the analysis, and reporting of urgent and routine samples.

Whilst regarding the assessment of process as the most direct approach to assessment of quality, Donabedian describes two other approaches, the assessment of *structure* and the assessment of *outcome*.

The concept of structure is used to embrace human, physical and financial resources. Structure as an assessable component of quality is readily understood in terms of appropriate numbers of staff, suitability of equipment, etc.

Outcome is used to mean a change in a patient's current and future health status as a result of a particular intervention, such as a course of treatment or the performance of a surgical procedure. Outcome is sometimes equated to the performance of a laboratory in external quality assessment schemes, but must encompass broader issues involved in clinical audit such as evaluating the choice of test or procedure in the context of diagnosis, prognosis or monitoring of disease and whether it had an appropriate effect on the healthcare outcome for an individual patient.

Chapters 5-8 deal with aspects of structure, such as organisation and management, staffing, buildings and equipment, and Chapter 11 with quality assurance, and evaluation or assessment of outcomes.

SOURCES OF STANDARDS

When preparing for accreditation it is not only important to think carefully about what a standard means, but also to think about the sources of information that supplement the standard. This information can come from many places and it is the intention in this section of the book to draw attention to these resources. The sources of standards are numerous and only a few examples are given in Figure 2.5. Others will be quoted where appropriate throughout the text.

It is often said that no accreditation scheme is truly voluntary. However, even in countries such as the United Kingdom, where as yet there is no legislation governing accreditation of laboratories, a standard or explanatory information associated with the standard will point to a requirement to comply with current legislation. For example CPA Standard C11 states 'There is a safe working environment in accordance with current legislation'.

International	• World Health Organisation (WHO) • International Organisation for Standardisation (ISO) • International Union of Pure and Applied Chemistry (IUPAC) • Organisation of Economic Co-operation & Development (OECD) • European Community (EC) • The joint European Standards Organisation (CEN/CENLAC)
National	• Government legislation, e.g. CLIA'88 [United States of America] • National Council for Clinical Laboratory Standards (NCCLS) [USA] • National accreditation schemes • Professional Societies • Management consultants • Patient groups
Local	• Local groups of professional organisations and local hospitals, particularly in clinical audit. • Purchaser / provider contracts.

Figure 2.5 Sources of standards

STANDARDS USED AS MAIN REFERENCES

There are certain quality and accreditation systems that are increasingly recognised as being of importance internationally, such as the ISO 9000 and EN 45000 series of standards and the OECD Principles of Good Laboratory Practice. The standards of the Laboratory Accreditation Program of the College of American Pathologists and of Clinical Pathology Accreditation (UK) Ltd are quoted as representative of systems derived from different traditions, well tested and tried in practice. Throughout this book where appropriate, the requirements of these standards with respect to a particular subject will be quoted at the relevant point. For example, the requirement in different quality and accreditation systems for a quality manual is shown in Figure 4.14.

Organisation	Title of the standard	Abbreviation
International Organisation for Standardisation (ISO)	ISO 9001:1994 Quality systems. Model for quality assurance in design, development, production, installation and servicing	**ISO 9001:1994**
The joint European Standards Organisation (CEN/CENLAC)	EN 45001:1989 General criteria for the operation of testing laboratories	**EN 45001:1989**
Organisation of Economic Co-operation and Development (OECD)	OECD Principles of Good Laboratory Practice (1981)	**OECD-GLP**
College of American Pathologists (CAP)	Standards for Laboratory Accreditation (1988 Edition)	**CAP-LAP**
Clinical Pathology Accreditation (UK) Ltd (CPA)	Accreditation Handbook-Standards and guidelines (1994)	**CPA(UK)Ltd**

Figure 2.6   Standards used as main references

The title of the standards, with names of the promulgating organisations, and the abbreviations used throughout the book are given in Figure 2.6, (addresses for the organisations are given in Appendix 1). The history and development of the organisations was given in Chapter 1. In this section the structure and content of the quality and accreditation systems will be outlined and the use of the word standard and/or its equivalents discussed.

ISO 9000 SERIES OF QUALITY SYSTEM STANDARDS (ISO)

The three standards in the ISO 9000 series represent 'distinct forms of quality systems requirements suitable for the purpose of a supplier (laboratory) wishing to demonstrate its capability, and for assessment of the capability of the supplier by external parties' (Figure 2.7).

The ISO 9001:1994 standard will be quoted throughout this book as it is considered that the activity of a pathology laboratory (see next chapter, Figure 3.1) includes design and development, as well as aspects of production, installation and servicing. If a laboratory is not undertaking design and development activities in relation to the services which it offers, then ISO 9002:1994 is a more appropriate standard.

ISO 9001	Quality systems - Model for quality assurance in design, development, production, installation and servicing.
	(To be used when conformance to specified requirements is to be assured by the supplier during design, development, production, installation and servicing - see Figure 2.8 for the clauses)
ISO 9002	Quality systems - Model for quality assurance in production, installation and servicing.
	(To be used when conformance to specified requirements is to be assured by the supplier during, production, installation and servicing - as ISO 9001 minus clause 4.4)
ISO 9003	Quality systems - Model for quality assurance in final inspection and test.
	(To be used when conformance to specified requirements is to be assured by the supplier solely at final inspection and test - as ISO 9001 minus clauses 4.3, 4.4, 4.6, 4.7, 4.9, 4.14, 4.17, 4.19)

Figure 2.7   The ISO 9000 series of quality systems standards

The alphanumeric identifier of the standard varies depending on the context in which the standard is used, ISO 9001:1994 being the international form, EN ISO 9001:1994 when adopted as a European standard and BS EN ISO 9001:1994 when used in the United Kingdom.

In international standards such as ISO 9001:1994 the whole document is termed a standard. The text of ISO 9001:1994 which enumerates the quality systems requirements uses the term 'provisions of this International Standard' in the same sense in which the word standard is used by CAP-LAP or CPA(UK)Ltd. These provisions are laid out in separate paragraphs or clauses and are presented in Figure 2.8. Unlike other standards referred to in this book, the ISO 9000 series of standards are intended for use in all situations which require a quality management system and are not limited in their application to laboratories. However, because of its industrial origins, the wording of the provisions will not at first sight appear to be relevant to the pathology laboratory. In Chapter 3, as part of 'preparing for accreditation', the provisions will be put in the context of a pathology laboratory.

In addition to these standards there is document ISO 9000-1:1994 providing guidance on which of the three quality systems standards is suitable for particular situations. Although it is intended that the standards should be used in their present form, there may be specific contractual situations which require the addition or deletion of certain quality system requirements and advice about this is given in ISO 9000-1. Other ISO documents such as ISO 8402:1994 'Quality management and quality assurance - Vocabulary' and ISO 10013:1995(E) 'Guidelines for developing quality manuals' will be introduced and discussed in appropriate sections of this book.

Clause number	Title of the clause (provision)
4.1	Management responsibility
4.2	Quality system
4.3	Contract review
4.4	Design control
4.5	Document and data control
4.6	Purchasing
4.7	Control of customer-supplied product
4.8	Product identification and traceability
4.9	Process control
4.10	Inspection and testing
4.11	Control of inspection, measuring and test equipment
4.12	Inspection and test status
4.13	Control of non conforming product
4.14	Corrective and preventive action
4.15	Handling, storage, packaging, preservation and delivery
4.16	Control of quality records
4.17	Internal quality audits
4.18	Training
4.19	Servicing
4.20	Statistical techniques

Figure 2.8   The provisions of ISO 9001:1994

EN 45000 STANDARDS (CEN/CENLAC)

The origin of the EN 45000 series of standards and their relationship to the ISO/IEC Guides was discussed in Chapter 1. Information on the series of standards covering testing, certification and accreditation is given in Figure 2.9. The first three standards EN 45001-EN 45003, define the three elements of an accreditation system, giving in EN 45001 the criteria for the acceptable operation of a testing laboratory, in EN 45002 the criteria for assessment or inspection of that laboratory, and in EN 45003 the criteria for the conduct of the accreditation body itself. As with the ISO 9000 standards, the whole of EN 45001:1989 'General criteria for the operation of testing laboratories' is regarded as a standard and the use of the word 'criteria' in the title can be interpreted in the same sense in which the word standard is used by CAP-LAP or CPA (UK) Ltd.

EN 45001	General criteria for the operation of testing laboratories.
EN 45002	General criteria for the assessment of testing laboratories.
EN 45003	General criteria for laboratory accreditation bodies.
EN 45011	General criteria for certification bodies operating product certification.
EN 45012	General criteria for certification bodies operating Quality System certification.
EN 45013	General criteria for certification bodies operating certification of personnel.
EN 45014	General criteria for suppliers' declaration of conformity.

Figure 2.9   The EN 45000 series of standards

In Section 5 'Technical competence' in EN 45001:1989, the criteria of the standard are enumerated under the section headings as given in Figure 2.10.

5 Technical competence

5.1	Management and organisation
5.2	Personnel
5.3	Premises and equipment

	5.3.1	Availability
	5.3.2	Premises and environment
	5.3.3	Equipment

5.4	Working procedures

	5.4.1	Test methods and procedures
	5.4.2	Quality System
	5.4.3	Test reports
	5.4.4	Records
	5.4.5	Handling of test samples or items
	5.4.6	Confidentiality and security
	5.4.7	Subcontracting

Figure 2.10   The criteria of the EN 45001:1989 standard

PRINCIPLES OF GOOD LABORATORY PRACTICE (OECD)

The history of the development of GLP was given in Chapter 1. When good laboratory practice becomes formalised it becomes known as 'Principles of Good Laboratory Practice' and the word *principle* here is being used in a similar sense to standard. In the OECD Principles of Good Laboratory Practice, the principles are grouped into the sections shown in Figure 2.11.

1.	Test facility organisation and personnel
2.	Quality Assurance programme
3.	Facilities
4.	Apparatus, material, and reagents
5.	Test systems
6.	Test and reference substances
7.	Standard Operating Procedures
8.	Performance of the study
9.	Reporting of study results
10.	Storage and retention of records and material

Figure 2.11   The principles of OECD-GLP

COLLEGE OF AMERICAN PATHOLOGISTS

In the College of American Pathologists laboratory accreditation program (CAP-LAP), there are five standards (see Figure 2.12). Each standard is then followed by an interpretation; these are comments which clarify what has to be undertaken to fulfil each standard. An example of these interpretative notes in relation to the role and responsibilities of a laboratory director is given in Chapter 5, Figure 5.5.

I	Director and personnel requirements.
II	Resources and facilities.
III	Quality assurance.
IV	Quality control.
V	Inspection requirements.

Figure 2.12   The standards of the CAP laboratory accreditation program

In addition to the interpretative notes there are an extensive series of checklists which have to be completed prior to the on-site inspection, and also for the mid-cycle self evaluation. There are checklists for General Laboratory, Haematology, Clinical Chemistry, Urinalysis, Clinical Toxicology/Therapeutic Drug Monitoring, Microbiology (including Bacteriology, Mycobacteriology, Mycology, Parasitology, and Virology), Transfusion Medicine, Diagnostic Immunology and Syphilis Serology, Nuclear Medicine (in vitro and radioimmunoassay procedures), Anatomic Pathology and Cytology, Clinical Histocompatibility, Flow Cytometry, and for a Limited Service Laboratory.

| | PHASE | QUESTION NUMBER | | CIRCLE ONE | |

Longitudinal process quality control procedures for individual instruments or inter-instrument comparisons may include;
A. use of preserved or stabilised whole blood controls,
B. retained patient specimens,
C. "moving average" monitoring of red cell indices, or
D. some combination of the above.

LAB

Does the laboratory use preserved or stabilised whole blood preparations for longitudinal process control?	0	02.2580	N/A	YES	NO

LAB

| Does the laboratory use retained, previously analyzed patient whole blood samples for longitudinal process control? | 0 | 02.2582 | N/A | YES | NO |

| Are an appropriate number of analyses of stabilized control or previously analyzed patients specimens performed and recorded on every shift of analyzer used? | II | 02.2585 | N/A | YES | NO |

NOTE: If stabilised control materials are used, they should preferably be obtained from more than one manufacturer and may be at different analytical levels (e.g., normal and high) Similarly, retained patient specimens should be of differing leukocyte, erythrocyte and platelet counts, as applicable

Figure 2.13   Section from the CAP-LAP checklist for quality control in haematology

A section from the Quality Control section of the 1996 Edition of the Inspection checklist for Haematology is shown in Figure 2.13. The Haematology inspection checklist contains 216 individual questions. When LAB appears against a question then only those questions have to be answered prior to submission of the application or reapplication. All other questions are answered by the inspector during the on-site inspection. Each question is assigned a 'phase' category, those in phase 0 are questions 'for information only', in phase I the questions 'represent items which are considered important in the management of an outstanding laboratory service', therefore, Phase I deficiencies should be corrected. Phase II questions 'represent items which are of a major importance and are essential to the management of a laboratory'. Phase II deficiencies are major defects and must be corrected before accreditation can be granted.

CLINICAL PATHOLOGY ACCREDITATION (UK) LTD

In the United Kingdom, the Clinical Pathology Accreditation system has 44 Standards and they are grouped together in six sections (Figure 2.14). Section A entitled 'Organisation and Administration' contains the standards dealing with the relationship

A	Organisation and Administration.
B	Staffing and Direction.
C	Facilities and Equipment.
D	Policies and Procedures.
E	Staff Development and Education.
F	Evaluation.

Figure 2.14 The sections of the CPA(UK)Ltd standards

between the laboratory and its host organisation; Section B 'Staffing and Direction' deals with staffing and management within the laboratory; Section C 'Facilities and Equipment' with the physical and environmental aspects of the laboratory and the equipment in that laboratory; Section D 'Policies and Procedures' details the requirements for the different processes taking place in the laboratory; and Section E 'Staff Development and Education' with making sure the staff have the on-going education and training to undertake the tasks required of them. Finally, standards in Section F 'Evaluation' are concerned with quality assurance and audit activities.

The standards are then followed by *guidelines* which, as with the word *interpretation* in the CAP scheme, aim to clarify the requirements of the standard. Forty-one of the 44 standards are common to the whole of pathology. One of the exceptions together with its guidelines is shown in Figure 2.15.

D14 In hospitals, a nominated consultant in the microbiology department is responsible for infection control

Guidelines:

1. There must be a written policy describing all aspects of infection control, and there must be an infection control committee of which a nominated consultant in microbiology must be a member*.

2. Hospital departments of Microbiology should support National/Regional reports of epidemiology of infection by regular reporting to Communicable Disease Surveillance Centre.

* Hospital Infection Control Working Group of the Department of Health and PHLS 'Hospital Infection Control: Guidance on the control of infection in hospitals' PHLS (1995)

Figure 2.15 CPA(UK)Ltd Section D Policies and Procedures - Standard D14

STANDARDS USED AS OTHER REFERENCES

In this section a brief background is given to other standards. It is not intended to be exhaustive and other material will be introduced throughout the book.

GOVERNMENT LEGISLATION

In the United States of America perhaps the most detailed example of standards being established in a regulatory context is the Final Rule published in the Federal Register Vol. 57 No. 40 on February 28th 1992 which implements the Clinical Laboratory Improvement Amendments of 1988 (CLIA'88). Set in very small type, it occupies one hundred and nine, three column pages. It describes in detail what is required of laboratories which perform tests at three levels of complexity, the so-called Waived tests, the Moderate complexity tests, and the High complexity tests.

The detailed requirements are given in subparts, conditions and standards. The subpart defines the issue, e.g. Subpart J Patient Test Management, condition is either general to the whole of Pathology or specific to a discipline, and the standard is the requirement for compliance. An example of part of the legislation and its structure is given in Figure 2.16. The subparts that refer to the major requirements of the legislation are:

- Participation in Proficiency testing
- Patient Test Management
- Quality Control, Personnel
- Quality assurance
- Inspection.

Subpart J - Patient test management for Moderate or High Complexity Testing or Both.

493.1101	Condition: Patient test management; moderate or high complexity, or both.
493.1103	Standard: Procedures for specimen submission and handling.
493.1105	Standard: Test requisition.
493.1107	Standard: Test records.
493.1109	Standard: Test report.
493.1111	Standard: Referral of specimens.

Figure 2.16 CLIA'88 subpart, condition and standard.

NATIONAL COUNCIL FOR CLINICAL LABORATORY STANDARDS

Although the National Council for Clinical Laboratory Standards (NCCLS) is a national body (USA) it does in fact collect opinion from its world-wide membership and its publications are very highly regarded throughout the world. It is a non-profit making, educational organisation that provides a communication forum for the development, promotion, and use of national and international standards. Founded in 1968 and accredited by the American National Standards Institute, it is based on the principle that voluntary consensus standards are essential for maintaining the performance of the clinical laboratory at the high level necessary for quality patient care. Its active membership is open to professional and clinical societies, manufacturers and suppliers of products for patient testing, and regulatory and scientific agencies of government in the Americas. Corresponding membership is open to laboratories and health care institutions worldwide.

NCCLS publications describe laboratory procedures, bench and reference methods, and evaluation protocols applicable in all the major laboratory disciplines. The consensus process, under which the publications are reviewed, consists of formal procedures describing the development of an NCCLS document and criteria for its acceptance as a clinical laboratory standard.

Most NCCLS documents are subject to three levels of consensus - proposed, tentative, and approved. The comments of laboratory users are essential to the consensus process. Anyone may submit a comment and all comments are addressed, according to the consensus process, by the NCCLS committee that wrote the document. Comments either result in a change to the document when published at the next consensus level, or the committee responds in an appendix to the document. Comments are especially important at the proposed level.

An NCCLS document is published as a standard, guideline, or committee report. A *standard* is a document developed through the consensus process and clearly identifies specific, essential requirements for materials, methods, or practices for use in an unmodified form. A standard may, in addition, contain discretionary elements, which are clearly identified. A *guideline* is a document developed through the consensus process and describing criteria for a general operating practice, procedure, or material for the clinical laboratory community. A guideline may be used as written or modified by the user to fit specific needs. Finally, *reports* are documents which have not been subjected to consensus review and are released by the Board of Directors.

Indication of the status of the NCCLS is shown by the CAP-LAP requirement in the interpretative notes to Standard IV Quality control, which says in reference to Procedure manuals, '(they) should follow a standard format and indicate sources, dates of adoption, and evidence of periodic review as described in the NCCLS *Clinical Laboratory Technical Procedure Manual - Second Edition; Approved Guideline (GP2-A2,1992)'*, Examples of NCCLS documents will be quoted throughout the book and the address is given in Appendix 1.

NATIONAL PATHOLOGY ACCREDITATION ADVISORY COUNCIL (AUSTRALIA)

The National Pathology Accreditation Advisory Council (NPAAC) of Australia has published a series of laboratory assessment checklists. In the introduction to these checklists it says 'The checklists are intended to be used by the person in charge…to inform himself/herself of the areas which are thought to be important in the maintenance of standards'. As with CAP-LAP there are checklists for all the main disciplines in pathology. The checklists present a series of questions, e.g. the section on Microscopes in 'The Laboratory Assessment Checklist - Microbiology Section (1987)' is shown in Figure 2.17.

In the introduction to the checklist the concept of categories of question is introduced. It states ' Not all the points covered in the Checklist are equally important, and an attempt has been made to indicate which of the three categories each question falls into. It will be noticed that many of the questions are posed in a way which implies a positive answer, and in general it is expected that acceptable laboratories will be able to give such answers

- possibly with some variation due to their particular circumstances. Other questions are marked with an asterisk (*) and this indicates that the requirements must be met, and a third category marked with a hatch (#) to indicate the type of information that may be required during the accreditation process' (see Figure 2.17).

```
        3.4   MICROSCOPES                                            CIRCLE ONE

             *3.4.1   Are there sufficient microscopes available
                      with oil-immersion objectives...............   Yes  No  N/A

              3.4.2   Are there sufficient 'plate' microscopes,
                      i.e. stereoscopic binocular lowpower ........   Yes  No  N/A

             *3.4.3   Are all microscopes clean and well maintained   Yes  No  N/A

             *3.4.4   Is the illumination adequate on all
                      microscopes.................................    Yes  No  N/A

              3.4.5   Is dark ground microscopy available.........    Yes  No  N/A

             #3.4.6   Is phase contrast available.................    Yes  No  N/A

             #3.4.7   Is polarised light available................    Yes  No  N/A

             #3.4.8   Is fluorescent microscopy available.........    Yes  No  N/A

              3.4.9   Are the hours of use of high energy light
                      sources recorded............................    Yes  No  N/A
```

Figure 2.17 NPAAC checklist for microbiology - microscopes.

In addition to checklists, the NPAAC publishes guidelines. One which is particularly appropriate to a country with such large distances between centres of population, has been prepared with the assistance of the International Air Transport Association (IATA) and is entitled 'Guidelines for the transportation of pathology specimens as regular commercial freight'.

FURTHER READING

Accreditation Handbook. Version 6.4 1996. Clinical Pathology Accreditation (UK) Ltd.

Clinical Laboratory Improvement Amendments of 1988; Final Rule. Federal Register Vol.52/No.40/Friday, 28 February 1992/Rules and Regulations.

Donabedian A. The Definition of Quality and approaches to its assessment. 1980. Health Administration Press, Ann Arbor, Michigan.

EN 45001:1989. General criteria for the operation of testing laboratories. European Committee for Standardization.

EN 45020:1993. Glossary of terms for Standardization and related activities. European Committee for Standardization.

Guidelines for Transportation of Pathology Specimens as regular commercial freight. Commonwealth Department of Health, National Pathology Accreditation Advisory Council 1987.

Inspection Checklist, Haematology. 1995.1 Section II, College of American Pathologists.

ISO 8402:1994 Quality Management and quality assurance - Vocabulary. International Organisation for Standardization.

ISO 9001:1994. Quality Systems - Model for quality assurance in design, development, production, installation and servicing. International Organization for Standardization.

Laboratory Assessment Checklist in Microbiology, Commonwealth Department of Health, National Pathology Accreditation Advisory Council 1987.

OECD Principles of Good Laboratory Practice. Annex II to Decision of the Council of 12 May 1981 (c(81)30 Final).

Standards for Laboratory Accreditation. College of American Pathologists - Laboratory Accreditation Program 1988 Edition (contents slightly edited for 1994).

Chapter 3

Preparing for accreditation

INTRODUCTION

This chapter discusses the first steps in preparing for accreditation, and provides an introduction to chapters 4-11. There are two fundamental issues to consider in preparing for accreditation, regardless of which scheme is being followed, what work needs to be done and who should undertake it?

Before discussing preparation for accreditation further, a definition of the term 'laboratory' is required. In general hospitals which serve a local population, the most common arrangement is that 'disciplines or departments' are managed as 'the pathology laboratory'. Within such a structure, individual disciplines or departments retain greater or lesser degrees of autonomy. There are many variations on such an arrangement and in particular the number of disciplines which may be represented. The laboratory also has a relationship with its parent body or host organisation which can hinder or facilitate the way in which it works and thus upon whether it may or may not be able to meet particular standards. The model which will be used in this book is shown in its simplest form as a 'family tree' in Figure 3.1.

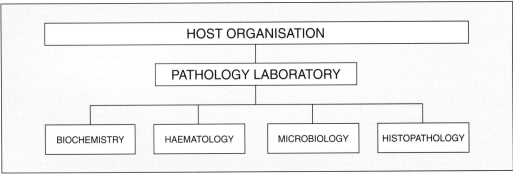

Figure 3.1   The pathology laboratory as a family tree.

Throughout the remaining chapters reference will be made to the Pathology Laboratory of St Elsewhere's Hospital Trust . This is a fictional entity and bears no relationship to any hospital laboratory either 'living or dead'. Further information about the laboratory and the services it provides can be found in Figure 5.15.

WHAT WORK NEEDS TO BE DONE?

Preparation for any scheme of accreditation requires both an analysis of the laboratory organisation and an investigation of what is already in existence particularly in terms of documentation. The analysis of the organisation of the laboratory can be undertaken in terms of where things are done, the structural or 'family tree' approach, and in terms of how things are done, the functional or 'type of activity' approach.

ORGANISATION OF THE LABORATORY

THE FAMILY TREE

As shown in Figure 3.2, the family tree model of the pathology laboratory shown in figure 3.1 can be developed further. Disciplines can be divided into work centres or sections, and within a work centre there are often a number of test sites.

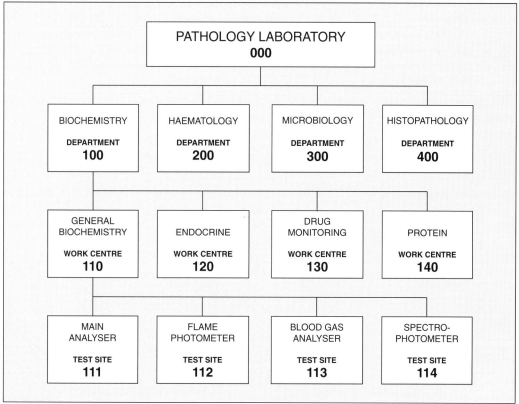

Figure 3.2   Departments, work centres and test sites

Pathology computer systems generally require that the different levels of organisation are identified by a numbering system. The first digit of a three digit number represents the department, the second the work centre or section, and the third the test site. When procedures are being written they can be numbered to indicate the level of organisation to which they apply. Such a system can be equally useful in a laboratory that is not computerised. Some laboratories may prefer to use letters instead of numbers or alternatively a combination of both letters and numbers. This organisational analysis is important as it enables activities that are valid across the whole of the laboratory to be distinguished from those limited in their application to a particular part of the laboratory. A written procedure for telephoning results might be adopted by all disciplines in the laboratory, whereas a laboratory procedure for blood culture would be specific to a particular work centre or test site.

The main benefit of the family tree approach is that it gives a logical way in which to organise the documentation of laboratory methods. If the accreditation system to be used is based on ISO 9001:1994 which requires the design of a quality management system, an analysis of the organisation will identify at what level procedures are required and allow the creation of a coherent system of documentation.

OPERATING PROCESSES AND SUPPORT ACTIVITIES

Having identified that the organisation of a laboratory can usefully be described in terms of a family tree, there is another equally important analysis and that is in terms of activities.

When considering the organisation of a laboratory it is useful to distinguish 'operating process activities' from 'support activities'. The regular maintenance of a piece of equipment is a support activity whereas staining slides for histopathological examination is an operating process activity. This division of activities within an organisation can be equated to the 'components of quality which can be assessed' described by Donabedian. Thus, the Donabedian concept of 'process' directly relates to operating process activities and 'structure' and 'outcome' equate to support activities (Figure 3.3).

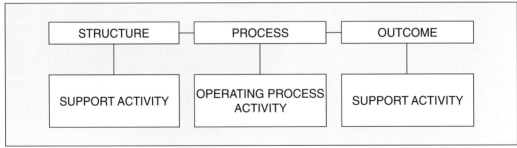

Figure 3.3   Relationship between components of quality and activities

The operating process activities mean everything that takes place from the initial decision to collect a specimen from a patient, to its transport, reception and analysis and to the reporting and interpretation. As shown in Figure 3.4 these operating processes are conveniently separated into preanalytical, analytical and postanalytical phases.

Description of the activities associated with the operating process in a pathology laboratory is unlikely to be contentious. However, which activities to regard as support activities is not so easy. Broadly speaking however, they are all activities associated with structure and outcome. Looking back at Figure 2.14, the CPA(UK)Ltd standards in section D Policies and Procedures are operating process activities, and they have their equivalents in other

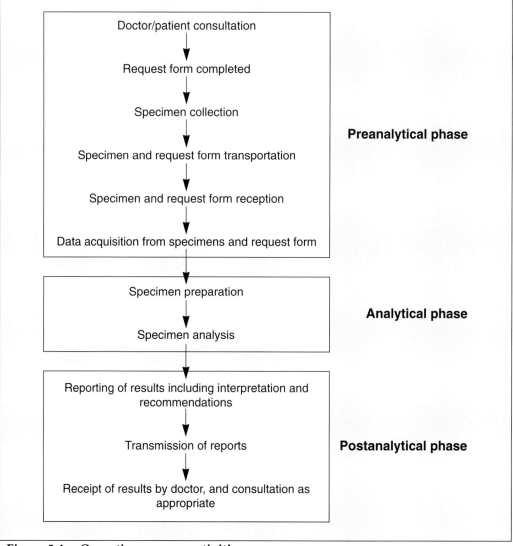

Figure 3.4   Operating process activities

schemes. CPA Sections A, B, C, E and F can be classified as support activities. In accreditation schemes with well-defined standards it is possible to associate a particular standard with a particular operating process activity and this can be good preparation both for understanding how standards equate to laboratory processes and devising an audit trail for the assessment or inspection of a laboratory.

Laboratories which have decided to seek accreditation using the ISO 9000 series of standards will have had to face the difficult task of interpreting and equating the clauses of the

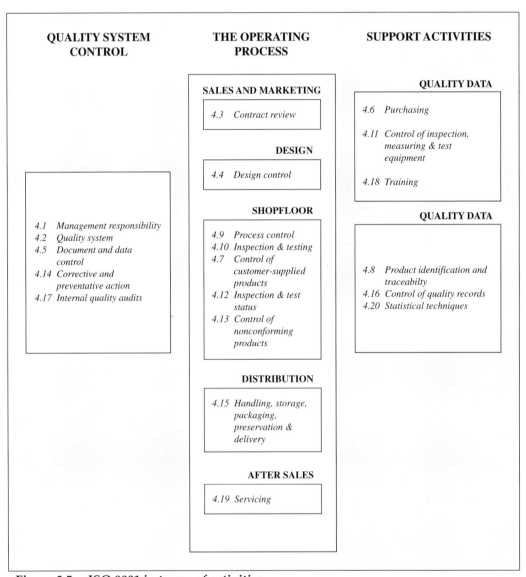

QUALITY SYSTEM CONTROL

4.1 Management responsibility
4.2 Quality system
4.5 Document and data control
4.14 Corrective and preventative action
4.17 Internal quality audits

THE OPERATING PROCESS

SALES AND MARKETING
4.3 Contract review

DESIGN
4.4 Design control

SHOPFLOOR
4.9 Process control
4.10 Inspection & testing
4.7 Control of customer-supplied products
4.12 Inspection & test status
4.13 Control of nonconforming products

DISTRIBUTION
4.15 Handling, storage, packaging, preservation & delivery

AFTER SALES
4.19 Servicing

SUPPORT ACTIVITIES

QUALITY DATA
4.6 Purchasing
4.11 Control of inspection, measuring & test equipment
4.18 Training

QUALITY DATA
4.8 Product identification and traceabilty
4.16 Control of quality records
4.20 Statistical techniques

Figure 3.5   ISO 9001 in terms of activities

standards to the requirements of a pathology laboratory. Jackson and Ashton, in 'Implementing Quality through BS 5750 (ISO 9000)' comment that "the arrangement of the twenty subclauses of the quality requirements of Section 4 of Part 1 is not user friendly". They rearrange the subclauses into an order which is more useful, and associate the clauses with 'The operating process', 'Quality system control' and 'Support activities'. The latter two groups could equally satisfactorily be described as support activities. Figure 3.5 is based upon Figure 2.1 of Jackson and Ashton's book but using clause titles from ISO 9001:1994. See also Figure 9.10 in Chapter 9 Operating process activities - preanalytical and postanalytical phases.

GETTING STARTED

ORGANISING THE WORK

If the clinical pathology laboratory as a whole decided to apply for accreditation then the first step is to form a working party for accreditation which should draw its membership from medical, scientific, technical and secretarial representatives of the different disciplines and be strongly supported by the Director of Pathology. As this is likely to be rather a large group then it should only meet every six to eight weeks and have as its main task designation and allocation of tasks and monitoring progress. Each discipline of pathology should have an individual who is responsible for progress in that discipline and they could chair the discipline working party. Figure 3.6 illustrates an ongoing record of progress by the biochemistry working group towards meeting standards.

The first thing to do is to collect information about what is already in place which might fulfil some of the requirements of the particular quality or accreditation system being addressed. In Chapter 4 there is a figure (Figure 4.1) which shows the hierarchy of documentation as a pyramid. If the pyramid is inverted with forms and records at the top, procedures and working instructions in the middle and policies at the bottom, it suggests a useful approach to discovering what is already in place. For example, collect together all the request forms in use and check if there is a written procedure for entering request data onto the laboratory computer. What is the policy for training new staff to use the computer? Collect together all forms used for recording tests done manually in Biochemistry. Do procedures exist for performance of manual tests? Do they refer to the forms in use?

The time allocated to the task should not be underestimated and the process will be greatly helped if a word processor and good secretarial support is available. It is estimated by many that at least eighteen months to two years will be required for the preparation stage prior to an application being made. The amount of work required by individual disciplines will vary greatly and those departments with a very broad test repertoire will need sympathetic support from those whose task is not so onerous. There are many benefits to be gained by a pathology department tackling the task together rather than as separate

ST ELSEWHERE'S HOSPITAL TRUST
Progress Report - Biochemistry Working Group (BWG) - CPA(UK)Ltd

Target date for submission of application 01/01/97   Date of report 20/05/96

Biochemistry Working Group Date	Action required	Action	Target date for current action	Target date for Standard to be met
Standard D7	**There is record of all reagents, calibration and quality control material**			**06/03/96**
22/11/95	*Preparation needs to continue, draft common procedure and forms for all sections*	*Section heads*	*06/03/96*	
09/10/95	*Each section head to be responsible for keeping records to common format?*	*BWG decision*	*22/11/95*	
Standard D8	**There is a written, signed and dated procedure for the performance of each test**			**08/08/96**
22/11/95	*Lists completed by all except Endocrinology. Urgent decision required as to format of revised procedures, see MP 000 002 by Pathology Working party.*	*Quality Officer*	*13/12/95*	
09/10/95	*Collect together all method sheets and forms used to record results. List all procedures required*	*Section heads*	*22/11/95*	

Figure 3.6   Mechanism for monitoring progress in the preparation for accreditation

disciplines. Many items requiring attention such as management, computing and communication procedures can be dealt with corporately, after all, no customer wants to receive a user handbook from each discipline! If a suitable individual can be seconded to the task to act as overall co-ordinator then this should progress matters swiftly providing the individual is good at enthusing other people and does not aggregate all the work to him / herself.

WHO SHOULD UNDERTAKE THE WORK?

It is an important principle that as many people as possible must be involved in the work and in appropriate parts of the work. Whereas it is entirely appropriate for the head of the laboratory to play a major role in preparing a user's handbook, it may not be appropriate for him/her to write laboratory procedures. Appropriate delegation of responsibility is important if staff are to have 'ownership' of the process, and an educational programme must explain the reasons for undertaking accreditation. For some staff knowing that their laboratory is in compliance with standards established by their peers may be motivation enough. For others it may come from knowing that certain contracts may only be open to accredited facilities.

In all accreditation systems there is a requirement for extensive documentation to be in place and the preparation of this documentation and its control is a major part of preparation for accreditation. Preparation is not a once only activity and a periodic review of all documentation is an essential requirement. These topics are explored further in the next chapter. Preparation for the structural components of quality are dealt with in Chapters 5-8, those of process in Chapters 9-10, and of outcome in Chapter 11.

THE APPLICATION

Most accreditation systems require a formal written application to be made to the accreditation body. Some systems require the completion of checklists and in some an application form has to be completed. For example in the case of CPA(UK)Ltd the application form to be completed is in two distinct sections, the first part requires details of the host organisation (hospital) and of the applicant pathology department. In the case of each department, details are required of the repertoire of tests and numbers performed each month, details of staffing, etc. The second section requires that the department formally records their compliance against each standard. Further information on the cycle of application, inspection and granting of accreditation for the different quality and accreditation systems will be given in Chapter 12. The Inspector calls!

FURTHER READING

Jackson P and Ashton D Implementing Quality Through BS 5750 (ISO9000), Kogan Paul London 1993.

Chapter 4

Policies, procedures, instructions and forms

NATURE OF DOCUMENTATION

The majority of standards in accreditation systems require documentary evidence to be available when the inspection takes place. This evidence can be very broad in nature and ranges from mission statements, quality manuals and detailed laboratory procedures, to minutes of meetings and work sheets, depending upon the particular accreditation system. The preparation of this documentation is perhaps the most lengthy and time consuming part of the accreditation process, but because of the evidential nature of many standards it is essential that it is undertaken in a systematic and structured way. Because of the wide range of documents involved it is useful to think of a hierarchy of documentation as shown in Figure 4.1

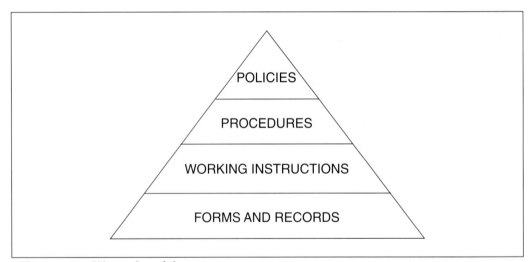

Figure 4.1   Hierarchy of documents

At the top of this hierarchy are the policies. A policy can be defined as 'setting out the commitment of an organisation to follow a particular course of action'. A pathology laboratory can have an overall policy statement which is inclusive of all aspects of the work of the laboratory or there can be a number of separate policies relating to different aspects of the laboratory's working. In many systems of accreditation it is a requirement to have a Quality Manual. This manual will contain the policy(ies) among other items of information (Chapter 5.15).

The second level in the hierarchy are the *procedures*. Procedures are the practical way in which policies are translated into action and are often called SOP's or standard operating procedures. It is 'a defined way of progressing a course of action or policy'. Policies can relate to management, quality assurance and laboratory methods etc. and procedures are needed which relate to the same areas.

The third level of documentation is *working instructions*. These are practical day to day instructions and, for example, might describe starting up or closing down a haematology analyser, a microbiology plate pouring machine, or a laboratory computer. Instructions can be embedded in a procedure or can be referred to in the procedure and published separately. In this presentation, working instructions will not be regarded as a separate type of document.

Finally, *forms and records*; it is important that recording any information or data such as patients results, quality control data or the result of an audit should be done on forms of an approved format and not on the back of an envelope. If the procedure requires some-thing to be recorded on a standard form it must be referred to in the procedure. The forms or records do not necessarily have to be created as 'hard copy' (a paper record) but a form can be completed, by anybody who has the correct access priority, on computer screens placed locally in the laboratory, in the consultants office etc. Data entered in this way and captured in a computer file would constitute a record. Nevertheless, this record has to be readily accessible for inspection. In a pathology laboratory, request forms and test reports are an example of such documentation and will be discussed further in Chapter 8.

An example of the hierarchy of documentation would be a policy stating that there should be a Health and Safety committee in the laboratory. A procedure would describe its membership, remit, conduct and the frequency of its meetings. The minutes of that committee would be a record. Part of the remit of the committee would be to carry out safety audits. A standard form should be used for recording such audits. Another exam-ple might be a policy requiring standard operating procedures for equipment in particu-lar sections of the laboratory, e.g. measurement of blood cell parameters using an auto-matic haematology analyser. The procedures produced as a result of such a policy would contain all the necessary information for conducting such measurements and might also refer to working instructions for starting the analyser and for closing it down. If the instrument had primary tube sampling and was interfaced to a laboratory computer then an example of a form would be a computer-generated work sheet to assist with checking in samples. Additionally, the computer file which holds the patient details and results should be regarded as a record. Such computer-held data needs to be as accessible on demand as any manually created paper record. The retention of these records and, in some accreditation systems, test samples is a matter of some importance and it is dictated by 'utility', 'need to know', and in some circumstances by the possibility of litigation.

The term 'protocol' is sometimes used interchangeably with the word 'procedure' and particularly when referring to clinical matters. However on the principle that it is best to use words which are readily understood, the term clinical procedures rather than clinical protocols will be used throughout this text.

ORGANISATION OF PROCEDURES, WORKING INSTRUCTIONS, RECORDS AND FORMS

THE QUALITY MANUAL

As we have seen, certain accreditation systems require a quality manual to be created but even if a system does not formally require a quality manual it is a good idea to develop one as it serves to introduce the policies and scope of the laboratory facility and to create an organisational structure for documentation. A quality manual can include all the procedures as well as policies or include policies only and make reference to the appropriate procedure manual. The purpose, structure and content of a quality manual will be dealt with in the next chapter on Organisation and Management but its relationship to procedures is discussed below.

PROCEDURE MANUALS

It is useful to see the quality manual as the introduction to all the procedures which have to be prepared as a result of the policies delineated in the quality manual. It may be desirable to put all procedures together in one procedure manual or to categorise them into separate manuals. Figure 4.2 shows such a hierarchy.

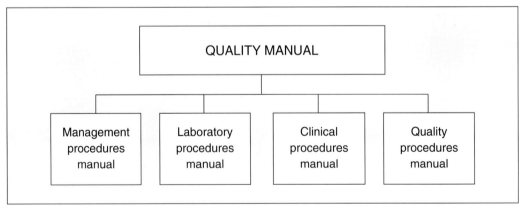

Figure 4.2   Organisation of manuals

Each manual should have an index and be regarded as volumes of the quality manual. Each of the manuals shown in Figure 4.2 would have a *master copy* and a known number of copies would be issued to appropriate places in the laboratory. Forms which are used in connection with a particular procedure will be referenced in that procedure and examples of the forms given in the appendix of the procedure.

In some disciplines, the laboratory procedures manual might be bulky and would need to be issued in parts to sections of the department. The titles of the manuals illustrated in Figure 4.2 are self-explanatory and with the exception of the laboratory procedures manual, which deals with operating process activities, all are to do with support activities. Contents of individual manuals will be dealt with in later chapters, management procedures in Chapters 5-8, laboratory procedures in Chapter 9-10, and quality assurance and clinical procedures in Chapter 11.

DOCUMENT PREPARATION AND CONTROL

PREPARATION AND CONTROL

The preparation of a document, whether it is a quality manual, procedure, working instructions or a form, should follow a particular course which is shown diagrammatically in Figure 4.3. If the document is a procedure or form it is best prepared or designed by the person who regularly carries out the procedure or is familiar with the particular activity e.g. scrutiny of results from external quality assessment schemes. The document is then subject to verification, in the case of a laboratory procedure preferably by a person who actually uses the procedure. There should be one person, in the laboratory or the discipline concerned, responsible for editing. In most cases this would be the designated Quality Manager. This person would also be responsible for ensuring that the style of individual documents was similar and, where appropriate, in compliance with GLP requirements.

It is useful to distinguish between *documents in preparation* and documents that have been *authorised and issued*. In the *draft editing and verification* stages, the documents are in preparation. During these stages any documents in circulation should be printed on **plain white paper** and are considered to be UNCONTROLLED documents. All copies that are *authorised and issued* officially should be marked with an edition number (the word 'edition' is used throughout this text rather than issue or version, as meaning 'one of a number of printings issued at separate times with alterations, amendments etc.') on the front page, signed by the author, and authorised by a responsible person (Figure 4.3). It can also be signed by the Quality Manager if one has been appointed. All such documents should be printed on **paper of a distinctive colour** and this paper should only be available for that purpose. These documents are CONTROLLED documents

If further copies are made of authorised and issued documents over and above those on the official circulation list, these must be printed on plain white paper.

Documents that have been withdrawn from use should be stored in archive manuals which parallel the manuals shown in Figure 4.2. It is a good rule to prepare as few copies as are absolutely necessary and to keep a record of the issue location in the index of the appropriate manual or in a master index of documents.

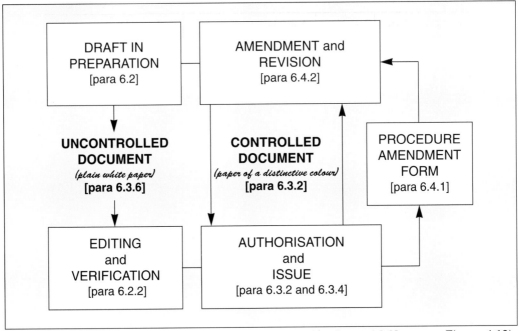

Figure 4.3   Preparation and control of documents (for [para 6.3.2] etc. see Figure 4.13)

When a procedure is in use, occasionally small typographical errors are discovered or minor amendments need to be made, and it is useful to attach to the back of the procedure a *procedure amendment form* on which a record is kept of such changes. This has to be under strict rules: (a) the amendment must be authorised by a section leader and must be considered minor, (b) the amendment must be underlined and an asterisk placed in the margin alongside the amendment, (c) ten or less amendments can be made before the procedure is revised, and (d) any major amendment must lead to an immediate full revision of the procedure and its re-issue as a subsequent edition or version. A minor amendment sheet is illustrated in Figure 4.4.

A minor amendment is an amendment that does not materially affect the operation of the procedure, such as correction of a spelling mistake or incorrect bolding. The figure for the

St Elsewhere's Hospital Trust	MF 000 022
PATHOLOGY	**Edition1** **Page 1/1**

PROCEDURE AMENDMENT FORM

Number	Date	Page No.	Amendment	Authorised by:
1				
2				
3				
4				
5				
6				
7				
8				
9				
10				

- The amendment must be authorised by the author of the procedure
- The amendment must be underlined and an asterisk written in the margin along side the change (*liquid paper must not be used*)
- Ten or less minor amendments can be made before the procedure is revised
- Major changes must result in the immediate review of the procedure

MANAGEMENT FORM

Figure 4.4   Procedure amendment form

number of amendments which can be made before revision is arbitrary but is intended to prevent the document becoming too untidy. Documents in use should maintain their quality, particularly with regard to legibility. Word processing packages have made the preparation of procedures relatively simple but care needs to be taken as they also enable alterations in an uncontrolled way.

If minor amendments are made they must be made in a specified manner and correction fluid must never be used. The correct and incorrect methods of making modifications are illustrated in Figure 4.5. In the example used, raw data is being modified, but the same rules apply to the modification of any authorised document being changed under the minor amendments procedure described above. Some authorities may not accept that minor amendments can be made in this way but, with care, it can provide a useful and controlled mechanism of making minor amendments.

Some authorities will not allow even minor changes to authorised and issued procedures and require that a new edition be issued whenever a change is made. The history of a document is important and in the case of a procedure, the 'history to date' can be kept with the current edition and must also form part of a master index of documents.

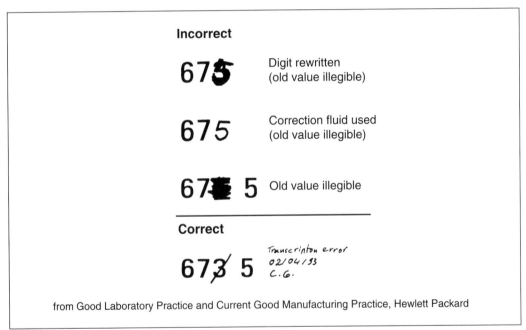

Figure 4.5   Modification of text or raw data

MASTER INDEX

The use of a *master index* is mentioned above in connection with the authorisation and issue of documents. It can either be hard copy or electronic media (e.g. a computer data base on disc) which enables a record to be kept of all documentation. In the ISO 9001:-

1994 Quality System 4.5 Document and data control 4.5.2 *Document data approval and issue* it states 'A master list or equivalent document control procedure identifying the current revision status of the documents shall be established and be readily available to preclude the use of invalid and/or obsolete documents'.

If the master index records include columns or fields for the 'date of issue' and the 'date of withdrawal' then it is possible to reconstruct an audit trail for the use of any procedure or form and also identify those documents in current use at any particular time. A suggested content of a master index record is show in Figure 4.6.

Item	Example
• Document code	*LP 100 013*
• Title of document	*Laboratory procedure for the measurement of urinary 5-OH Indole acetic acid*
• Edition	*3.0*
• Issue date	*29-May-96*
• Withdrawal date	*n/a*
• Total copies	*2*
• Department	*Clinical Biochemistry*
• Location 1	*Master copy (Quality Manager's Office)*
2	*Work centre 120 (Endocrine Laboratory)*
etc.	

Figure 4.6   Content of master index record

DOCUMENT IDENTIFICATION, FORMAT AND CONTENT

IDENTIFICATION

Individual documents need to have some unique identification code and, bearing in mind that most word processing packages have a fixed number of characters with which to name files or documents, a definite procedure needs to be adopted.

For example Microsoft® Word for Windows™, limits the filename to a maximum of eight characters with one to three characters for the filename extension (abcdefgh.doc). Any characters can be used except spaces and the following characters * ? : [ ] + = \ / |< >.

Different systems can be adopted using eight digits and some examples with explanations are given in Figure 4.7. The system shown uses the first two digits to identify the type of document, e.g. laboratory procedure or laboratory form etc. Up to six of the remaining digits can be used in any alpha numeric combination giving overall a unique eight digit identifier. This eight digit system for a pathology laboratory is further developed in Figure 4.13.

FIRST TWO DIGIT CODES

qm	quality manual
mp	management procedure
mf	management form
lp	laboratory procedure
lf	laboratory form
cp	clinical procedure
cf	clinical form
qp	quality procedure
qf	quality form

EIGHT DIGIT CODES

lp5iaa03.doc	laboratory procedure for the measurement of urinary **5** - OH indole acetic acid edition **03**
lp013e03.doc	laboratory procedure for procedure **013 e**dition **03** (The measurement of urinary 5-OH Indole acetic acid)
lp100013.doc	laboratory procedure for biochemistry **100** procedure **013** (The measurement of urinary 5-OH Indole acetic acid)

Figure 4.7   Document identification

FORMAT

Each page of a document whether it is a procedure, working instructions, or a form needs to contain certain information. The purpose of this information is to be able to identify a particular page as being page x of y pages coming from a particular document which belongs to a particular organisation.

There are a number of features in word processing packages that enable documents to be well designed and have features added to their text automatically and under control of the document creation process. The so-called header and footer facility allows information to be automatically printed on each page of a document and the page number to be incremented automatically. Figure 4.8 illustrates the use of the *header* and *footer* facility at

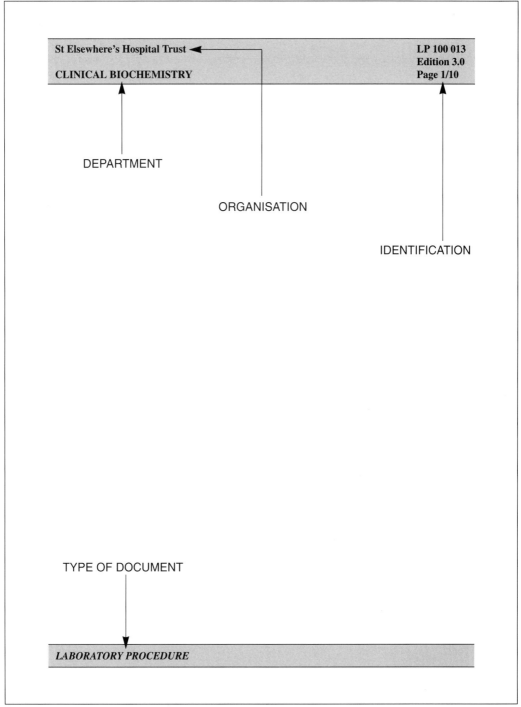

Figure 4.8   Use of the header and footer facility

St Elsewhere's Hospital Trust. The left-hand side of the *header* shows the name of the host organisation, St Elsewhere's Hospital Trust, and the department preparing the document (the case that is given is for Biochemistry but could alternatively be Pathology or any other discipline of pathology). The right-hand side of the *header* gives the document identification code, LP 100 013, the edition number 3.0, and the page number e.g. 1/10. The *footer* indicates the procedure manual to which the document belongs, and whether the document is a procedure or form. In addition to the identification of individual pages, a procedure must have a front page on which certain information is displayed. Different authorities have different views as to what should be included but Figure 4.9 gives an example.

- A descriptive title and indication of the SOP's position in the total collection

- Date when the SOP becomes operative

- The edition number and a statement that this edition replaces an early edition from an early date

- The exact distribution of the SOP

- The name and signature of the person responsible for writing the SOP

- The name and signature of the person responsible for authorising the SOP

- In some contexts the purpose of the SOP

modified from Good Laboratory and Clinical Practices
Edited by Carson PA and Dent N J (1990)

Figure 4.9   Front page information for an SOP

The descriptive title should indicate clearly the purpose of the procedure and a unique identification code indicates the SOP's position in the total collection. The edition number is important, and information as to which edition was replaced and the date. The operative date of the current edition will assist when audit, for example of internal quality control or external quality assessment data, is undertaken. Some laboratories include a review date and this is included in the example given (Figure 4.10).

The exact location of the procedure indicates where it is used in the organisation. The analysis of the organisation given in Figure 3.2 indicates how the location for laboratory procedures is derived. Of the information printed in the body of the front page a number of items can be drawn automatically from the file/summary information which can be recorded when a file (document) is being created in Microsoft® Word for Windows™. Figure 4.10 illustrates a sample front page.

As mentioned earlier, the history of an SOP is important and this can be either displayed on the first page or form the second history page. An example of such a history page is given in Figure 4.11.

| St Elsewhere's Hospital Trust

CLINICAL BIOCHEMISTRY | LP 100 057
Edition 5.0
Page 1/7 |

MEASUREMENT OF SERUM CK-MB CONCENTRATION

EDITION No:	*Edition 5.0*
OPERATIVE DATE:	*21-Jun-95*
REVIEW DATE:	*21-Jun-96*
REPLACES:	*Edition 4 19-Sep-94*
LOCATION:	*Work Centre 110 General Biochemistry* *Test site 114 Spectrophotometry*
AUTHOR: signature: date:	*David Burnett*
AUTHORISED BY: signature: date:	*John Qualimann*
COPY No.	*2/2*

LABORATORY PROCEDURE

Figure 4.10   Sample front page for a standard operating procedure

St Elsewhere's Hospital Trust	LP 100 057
	Edition 5.0
CLINICAL BIOCHEMISTRY	Page 2/7

HISTORY PAGE

Edition No	Date	Comment
1	17-Aug-93	
2	03-Jun-94	Amendment to kit insert.
3	28-Jul-94	Edition 2 reviewed. Addition of appendix 2 (establishment of internal means and ranges for ABC quality controls).
4	19-Sep-94	Replaces Edition 3, updating sections 4.6 and 4.7 due to replacement of computer interfaced to the ABC spectrophotometer.
5	21-Jun-95	Replaces Edition 4, updates ABC internal quality control ranges.

CIRCULATION LIST

Copy No	Location	Name	Signature
1	000 Quality Manager	John Qualiman	
2	100 Head of Biochemistry		
3	110 General Biochemistry, Work Centre Leader		

LABORATORY PROCEDURE

Figure 4.11 Example of an SOP history page

DOCUMENT CONTENT

The preceding paragraphs deal with the information which should appear on each page of any document and with the front and history pages of a procedure. The content of the body of a document will vary in accordance with the type of document. Most forms will be single pages with a fixed format, e.g. Figure 4.4. Procedures should have a general format which is illustrated in Figure 4.12 below.

1.0	Purpose and Scope
2.0	Responsibility
3.0	References
4.0	Definitions
5.0	Documentation
6.0	Action and methods

Figure 4.12   Main headings for the content of a procedure

The sort of material included under these headings is illustrated in Procedure for Document Preparation and Control (Figure 4.13). Purpose and Scope may refer to the implementation of a particular policy or, in the case of laboratory operating activity procedures, for the particular activity. Responsibility defines who is responsible for implementation of the procedure and to whom they report. Under the Reference section, appropriate source material can be quoted, and under Definitions any words which have a specific interpretation may be defined. Documentation refers to any forms used in the implementation of the procedure, and finally the section Action and Methods gives the content of the procedure.

AN SOP FOR PREPARING SOP'S

Many laboratories have a standard operating procedure for preparing SOP's. This is perhaps one of the most important of all laboratory documents and it may be preferable to expand its scope and call it a 'Procedure for document preparation and control'. A model for St Elsewhere's pathology laboratory is shown in Figure 4.13.

St Elsewhere's Hospital Trust	MP 000 002
	Edition 1
PATHOLOGY	Page 1/11

PROCEDURE FOR THE PREPARATION
AND CONTROL OF DOCUMENTS

EDITION No:	*Edition 1*
OPERATIVE DATE:	*13-May-95*
REVIEW DATE:	*13-May-96*
REPLACES:	*n/a*
LOCATION:	*000 Quality Assurance Unit*
AUTHOR: signature: date:	*John Qualimann*
AUTHORISED BY: signature: date:	*Director of Pathology*
COPY No.	*1/6*

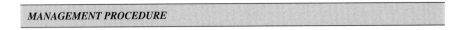

MANAGEMENT PROCEDURE

Figure 4.13 A model procedure for document preparation and control

St Elsewhere's Hospital Trust	MP 000 002
PATHOLOGY	Edition 1
	Page 2/11

HISTORY PAGE

Edition No	Date	Comment
1	13-May-95	
2		
3		
4		
5		

CIRCULATION LIST

Copy No	Post	Name	Signature
1	Quality Manager		
2	Director of Pathology		
3	Head of Biochemistry		
4	Head of Haematology		
5	Head of Microbiology		
6	Head of Histopathology		

MANAGEMENT PROCEDURE

Figure 4.13   A model procedure for document preparation and control (cont.)

St Elsewhere's Hospital Trust	MP 000 002
	Edition 1
PATHOLOGY	Page 3/11

TABLE OF CONTENTS

MANAGEMENT PROCEDURE

Figure 4.13   A model procedure for document preparation and control (cont.)

St Elsewhere's Hospital Trust	MP 000 002
	Edition 1
PATHOLOGY	Page 4/11

1 PURPOSE AND SCOPE

To define the procedure for preparation and control of all documents, including the Quality Manual, procedures and forms. (QM 000 001).

2 RESPONSIBILITY

2.1 THE QUALITY MANAGER

The Quality Manager is responsible to the Director of Pathology for the implementation of this procedure (see page 7 of the quality manual for the management structure of pathology).

2.2 THE QUALITY ASSURANCE UNIT

The quality manager will work closely with members of the quality assurance unit and other appropriate members of staff in carrying out paragraph 2.1.

3 REFERENCES

ISO 10013:1995(E) Guidelines for developing quality manuals.
LP 000 001 Procedure for preparation of procedures for operating process activities.

4 DEFINITIONS

Quality manager: person appointed to be in charge of the Quality Assurance Unit of the laboratory.
Responsible manager: persons responsible for overseeing the preparation and control of documentation in a particular area of the organisation.
Document: refers to any manual procedure or form prepared using this procedure.
Author: the person responsible for the preparation of any document.
Authorisation: the process of final checking, prior to issue, by an appropriate manager.
Operating process activities: activities directly involved in receipt, registration, processing and reporting on samples received.
Minor amendment: an amendment which does not materially affect the operation of the procedure e.g. spelling mistake or incorrect emboldening.
Non-conformance: failure to achieve a standard.

5 DOCUMENTATION

MF 000 001 Procedure amendment form
MF 000 002 Document circulation form

MANAGEMENT PROCEDURE

Figure 4.13   A model procedure for document preparation and control (cont.)

St Elsewhere's Hospital Trust	MP 000 002
	Edition 1
PATHOLOGY	**Page 5/11**

6 ACTIONS AND METHODS

6.1 DOCUMENT ORGANISATION

6.1.1 THE QUALITY MANUAL

The Quality Manual will be common to all departments in the Pathology Laboratory and will be held in a WHITE ring binder.

6.1.2 PROCEDURE MANUALS

The procedure manuals throughout the Pathology Laboratory will have common colour coding for the ring binders.

- Management procedure manuals   GREEN
- Laboratory procedure manuals   BLUE
- Clinical procedure manuals   YELLOW
- Quality procedure manuals   RED

The procedure manuals in each department will have some documents common to the whole of pathology and some specific to a particular department.

6.1.3 LABORATORY PROCEDURE MANUALS

Laboratory procedure manuals may be issued in a number of separate parts relating to the sections of a department.

6.2 DOCUMENT PREPARATION

6.2.1 RESPONSIBILITY

The Director of Pathology and the Heads of Department are responsible for requesting the preparation of documentation.

All documents will be written by those staff who are directly concerned with the area of work covered in the documentation.

6.2.2 EDITING AND VERIFICATION

All documents in preparation will have the words DOCUMENT IN PREPARATION on the front page immediately below the title. The authorisation panel (paragraph 6.3.2) will be incomplete and in particular have no authorising signatures or copy numbers. It is therefore an UNCON-TROLLED DOCUMENT (paragraph 6.3.6).

After preparation and before issue the documents will be verified for practical use by a member of staff involved in that area of work who did not prepare the document in question.

Editing for clarity, accuracy, suitability and proper structure should be done by a responsible man-ager before submission for authorisation (paragraph 6.3.2)

MANAGEMENT PROCEDURE

Figure 4.13   A model procedure for document preparation and control (cont.)

6.2.3 IDENTIFICATION AND FORMAT
6.2.3.1 Header and Footer
All document will carry a header and footer which will carry information as shown in this document,

- Institution (header - first top left).
- Department (header - second top left).
- Identification data (header - top right) which includes:
  * An eight digit identification code which is identical to the word processing file name minus the extension (.DOC in the case of Microsoft® Word for Windows™ except that the spaces are inserted after the first two and five digits (see paragraph 6.2.3.2)
  * Edition No.
  * Actual page/total number of pages.
- Type of document (footer - bottom left).

6.2.3.2 Identification Code
The structure of the eight digit identification code is as follows:

- The first two digits give the type of document (see below for codes).
- The next three contain the department (see below for list). Thus 200 would apply to the whole of Haematology etc.
- The final three digits are numerical and represent the number of the particular procedure
  e.g. this document numbered MP 000 002 = Management procedure for document preparation and control in the pathology laboratory.

Type of document and department are coded as shown below.

XX 000 000

TYPE of DOCUMENT	DEPARTMENT	PROCEDURE NUMBER
MP = Management Procedure **MF** = Management Form **LP** = Laboratory Procedure **LF** = Laboratory Form **CP** = Clinical Procedure **CF** = Clinical Form **QP** = Quality Procedure **QF** = Quality Form	000 = Pathology 100 = Biochemistry 200 = Haematology 300 = Microbiology 400 = Histopathology The second and third digit can be used to denote work centre and test site level e.g. 110 General Biochemistry 　　　111 Main Analyser	Three digit number starting from 001 within each document/department group e.g. LP 100 001 etc. Forms associated with the above procedure, move the right hand digit one position and number 1-9 e.g. LF 100 011

MANAGEMENT PROCEDURE

Figure 4.13   A model procedure for document preparation and control (cont.)

St Elsewhere's Hospital Trust	MP 000 002
PATHOLOGY	Edition 1 Page 7/11

6.2.4 CONTENT

6.2.4.1 Front page

The front page will include the title of the procedure and document control data (paragraph 6.3.2). This is not applicable to forms.

6.2.4.2 History and Distribution page

(Not applicable to forms)

6.2.4.3 Table of Contents

If the document is lengthy then it is valuable to include a contents page.

6.2.4.4 The remaining content for a procedure

The remaining content for a procedure is structured as in this procedure into the following sections:

1. PURPOSE AND SCOPE
2. RESPONSIBILITY
3. REFERENCES
4. DEFINITIONS
5. DOCUMENTATION
6. ACTION AND METHODS (this section can be variable depending on the purpose of the procedure, e.g. operating process activities, or support functions)

6.2.4.5 The remaining content of the Quality Manual

The remaining content of the Quality Manual is structured into the following sections,

SCOPE AND FIELD OF APPLICATION (on title page under title)
TABLE OF CONTENTS
0. INTRODUCTION TO THE ORGANISATION AND THE QUALITY MANUAL
1. THE QUALITY POLICY
2. DESCRIPTION OF THE ORGANISATION, RESPONSIBILITIES AND AUTHORITIES
3. DESCRIPTION OF THE ELEMENTS OF THE QUALITY SYSTEM AND ANY REFERENCES TO DOCUMENTED QUALITY SYSTEM PROCEDURES
4. DEFINITIONS SECTION, IF APPROPRIATE
5. GUIDE TO THE QUALITY MANUAL, IF APPROPRIATE
6. APPENDIX FOR SUPPORTIVE DATA

MANAGEMENT PROCEDURE

Figure 4.13   A model procedure for document preparation and control (cont.)

St Elsewhere's Hospital Trust	MP 000 002
	Edition 1
PATHOLOGY	Page 8/11

6.2.5 DOCUMENT MASTER INDEX

6.2.5.1 A Data Base (Microsoft Access$_{TM}$ file, MSTINDEX.MDB)

A data base of all the procedures is kept on computer file as a Master Index. Details kept on the master index are: -

- Document code
- Title of the document
- Edition
- Issue date
- Withdrawal date

- Total copies
- Department
- Location 1
- Location 2
- Location 3

6.2.5.2 Data deletion

No data will ever be deleted from this index. When a document is withdrawn from use the withdrawal date field in the master index will be completed to indicate that the document has been withdrawn from use (see paragraph 6.3.5) and kept in the Document archive library.

6.2.5.3 Listings from the Master index

The master index is used to produce a listing of the procedures relevant to particular procedure manuals. These lists will serve to create the Contents page of the appropriate manual.

6.3 DOCUMENT CONTROL

6.3.1 RESPONSIBILITY

The Director of Pathology is responsible for authorising the Quality Manual and Pathology Laboratory (000) documents, and the Heads of Department or other nominated responsible managers are responsible for authorising documents pertaining to their departments.

The document is then given to the Quality Manager for final approval. The authorisation data will then be added to the authorisation panel described in paragraph 6.3.2.

MANAGEMENT PROCEDURE

Figure 4.13 A model procedure for document preparation and control (cont.)

St Elsewhere's Hospital Trust	MP 000 002
	Edition 1
PATHOLOGY	Page 9/11

6.3.2 AUTHORISATION

When the COPY No. has been added to the authorisation panel (shown below) and the copies for issue signed by the author and the nominated responsible manager (paragraph 6.3.1), it is then a CONTROLLED document ready for issue (paragraph 6.3.4) and an entry can be made in the Master Index (paragraph 6.2.5). All CONTROLLED Documents (Quality Manual and Procedures but not forms) will be printed on **pink paper.**

EDITION No:	*Edition 1*
OPERATIVE DATE:	*31-May-95*
REVIEW DATE:	*31-May-96*
REPLACES:	*n/a*
LOCATION:	*000 Quality Assurance Unit* *100 Biochemistry*
AUTHOR: signature: date:	*John Qualimann*
AUTHORISED BY: signature: date:	*Director of Pathology*
COPY No.	*1/6*

6.3.3 COPIES

Each document (this excludes forms) will have at least two authorised copies, one to be kept in the Document Library (paragraph 6.3.5) and one in the relevant work area as part of the appropriate procedure manual. The total number of copies will depend on the content of the document. A copy of each Pathology document will be issued to each department or discipline for ready reference. The Document Master Index (paragraph 6.2.5) will record the location of copies.

MANAGEMENT PROCEDURE

Figure 4.13   A model procedure for document preparation and control (cont.)

St Elsewhere's Hospital Trust	MP 000 002
	Edition 1
PATHOLOGY	Page 10/11

6.3.4 ISSUE

When any new document or new edition of a document is issued it is essential that all relevant members of staff are made aware of its existence and content. It is the responsibility of the appropriate authorising person (paragraph 6.3.1) to ensure this.

To facilitate awareness, a circulation list (MF 000 021) should be issued for the document and circulated with a copy of the document. Those members of staff who need to be aware of the changes should be highlighted. All members on the circulation list should sign and date (DD-MMM-YY) it to show that they have read and understood the changes to a new edition or the contents of a new document, and the completed list stored with the appropriate procedure in the Document library.

6.3.5 REMOVAL OF REDUNDANT DOCUMENTS

When a new revision of a document has been authorised it will be the responsibility of the authorising manager to ensure that all redundant copies are removed from use. All library copies will be kept as a record of change. The withdrawal date should be entered in the Master Document Index.

Library copies should never be used as working documents. They are kept in the archive section of the Document library to facilitate retrospective audit.

6.3.6 UNAUTHORISED DOCUMENTS

Any document which is either unauthorised or a photocopy made for a third party is deemed to be unofficial. Documents being validated by trial will have the words 'DOCUMENT IN PREPARATION' under the title on the front page. All such documents are classified UNCONTROLLED DOCUMENT and are printed on white paper. Uncontrolled documents will not be updated.

6.4 DOCUMENT CHANGES

6.4.1 INITIATION OF AMENDMENTS

Any member of staff can suggest changes to controlled documents. Suggestions will be reviewed by the responsible manager.

If the amendment is considered by the responsible manager to be minor, then the change can be written on the procedure and the change recorded on the Procedure amendment form (MF 000 022). Such minor changes are subject to the rules outlined on the amendment form.

6.4.2 AMENDMENT AND REVISION

If the amendment is considered to be a major procedural change or is the tenth minor change then the document should be amended by the author or responsible manager.

After the amended document has been authorised (paragraph 6.3.2) and appropriate changes made to the history page of the document, a new entry should be made in the Master Index (paragraph 6.2.5), which should be reissued as a controlled document, Edition 2 (paragraph 6.3.4).

The amendments must be marked to show that they have changed from the previous edition.

MANAGEMENT PROCEDURE

Figure 4.13   A model procedure for document preparation and control (cont.)

6.5 COMPUTER DISK STORAGE

All files will be kept on an appropriately labelled computer disk by the Quality Manager.
For safety all files must have three copies. One on the hard disk, one on a disc working copy and a third on a disk which is to be kept in a protected area. The copy in the protected area will be updated as frequently as possible.

6.6 PRODUCT LIABILITY

6.6.1 MANUFACTURER'S METHOD SHEETS

In order that manufacturer's retain their legal obligations for product liability any proprietary method sheets which are supplied will be strictly adhered to. The original or a photocopy of the unaltered manufacturer's method sheet will form part of the laboratory procedure.

6.6.2 CHANGE TO MANUFACTURER'S METHOD

If there is a deviation from the manufacturer's method (e.g. performing single instead of duplicate tests) then the procedure will be rewritten as a complete laboratory procedure with no manufacturer's method sheet included.

Note: The manufacturer is no longer responsible under the obligations for liability.

6.7 DOCUMENTATION AUDIT

6.7.1 AUDIT

At regular intervals (see QP 000 001) the Quality Manager will instigate document audit to ensure they do not contain non-conformances. Specific attention will be paid to the following:

- All documents must be authorised (paragraph 6.3.2).
- All documents must be valid and contain no major hand-written changes. If changes are made the Procedure amendment form (MF 000 022) must be completed and attached to the procedure.
- All documents must be in the correct section of the laboratory and filed correctly.

The result of such audits will be recorded and discussed at meetings of the Quality Assurance Unit.

6.7.2 NON-CONFORMANCE

Any document which either fails audit or has been proved to be inaccurate will be amended and reissued by the responsible manager. All non-conforming copies except the Document library copy will be removed.

MANAGEMENT PROCEDURE

Figure 4.13   A model procedure for document preparation and control (cont.)

REQUIREMENTS FOR DOCUMENTATION

QUALITY MANUAL

The requirements for a Quality Manual in quality and accreditation systems are shown in Figure 4.14. It can be seen that only ISO 9001:1994 and EN 45001:1989 specify the requirement for a Quality Manual.

System	Quality Manual
ISO 9001:1994	**4 Quality system requirements** **4.2 Quality system** **4.2.1** *General* '.........The supplier shall provide a quality manual covering the requirements of this International Standard. The Quality Manual shall include or make reference to the quality system procedures and outline the structure of the documentation used in the quality system'.
EN 45001:1989	**5 Technical competence** **5.4 Working procedures** **5.4.2** *Quality system* ....The elements of this system shall be documented in a Quality Manual which is available for use by the laboratory personnel. The Quality Manual shall be maintained current by a nominated responsible member of the laboratory personnel.'
OECD - GLP	**2. Quality Assurance Programme** **2.1 General (1)** *No formal requirement but documentation of the quality assurance programme is required* ' The test facility should have a documented quality assurance programme...'
CAP - LAP	**Standard III Quality assurance** *'No formal requirement but the interpretation of* **Standard III** *says*, 'There shall be a written description of the program which, where applicable, shall be integrated with the institution's quality assurance program'.
CPA(UK)Ltd	**A Organisation and Administration** *No formal requirement but* **Standard A1** *states* 'There is a document to describe the organisation, scope and strategy of the applicant department and its satellite services'. (see also Figure 4.15).

Figure 4.14 Requirements for a quality manual

PROCEDURES AND OTHER DOCUMENTATION

The requirements for written procedures and other documentation are shown in Figure 4.15.

System	Procedures and other documentation
ISO 9001:1994	**4 Quality system requirements** **4.2 Quality system** **4.2.2 *Quality system procedures*** 'The supplier shall a) prepare documented procedures consistent with the requirements of this International Standard and the supplier's stated quality policy; ' **4.2.3 *Quality planning*** *Reference is made to another form of documentation called '**quality plans**' which will be mentioned in Chapter 11, but more information can be found in the references at the end of this chapter.*
EN 45001:1989	**5 Technical competence** **5.4 Working procedures** **5.4.1 *Test methods and procedures*** 'The testing laboratory shall have adequate documented instructions on the use and operation of all relevant equipment, on handling and preparation of test items (where applicable), and on standard testing techniques........All instructions, standards, manuals and reference data........ shall be maintained up-to-date and be readily available to personnel'.
OECD - GLP	**7. Standard operating procedures** **7.1 General** **(1)** 'A test facility should have written Standard Operating Procedures approved by management that are intended to ensure the quality and integrity of the data generated in the course of the study'. *Reference is also made to two other types of document which are unique and particular to GLP. A **study plan** - means a document which defines the entire scope of a study, (a study means an experiment or set of experiments in which a test substance is examined to obtain data on its properties and/or its safety with respect to human health and the environment) and a **final report** which is the document prepared at the conclusion of a study. The required content of both study plans and final reports are detailed in parts **8** and **9** of the GLP principles.*
CAP - LAP	**Standard IV Quality control** *The interpretative notes say* 'Procedure manuals should follow a standard format and indicate sources, dates of adoption and evidence of periodic review as described in the NCCLS Clinical Laboratory Technical Procedure Manual - 2nd edition; Approved Guideline (GP2-A2, 1992)'.
CPA(UK)Ltd	**D Policies and Procedures** *In the guidelines to* **Standard D1** *it says* 'In collaboration with service users, departmental policies, procedures and repertoire are fully documented in a readable manageable form and contain comprehensive information about the availability of clinical advice and the content and limitations of the service.' *This is similar to a requirement for quality and procedure manuals.*

Figure 4.15   Requirements for procedures and other documentation

STORAGE AND RETENTION OF DOCUMENTS AND SPECIMENS

All accreditation systems stipulate some requirements as to the storage and retention of documents and specimens. ISO 9001:1994 being a quality standard simply refers to retention and storage of quality records, whereas the laboratory focused standards refer to the retention of a number of distinct items which will vary depending upon the nature of the work being undertaken. The most comprehensive recommendations to be made in the clinical pathology field are to be found in a recent report from a Working Party of the Royal College of Pathologists entitled 'The Retention and Storage of Pathological Records and Archives' (see Appendix 3). Regulatory authorities, accreditation systems or individual pathologists in different countries may have differing views on how long records should be kept, but this publication is also valuable in detailing the nature and range of documents and specimen material to be considered. The times quoted for retention and storage are the recommended minimum times. Some recommendations, such as the requirement that internal quality control records should be kept permanently, may be seen as controversial. A distinction is drawn between Clinical and Diagnostic Records and Reports on the one hand and Laboratory Records such as Reports, Documentation and Specimens on the other hand. It points out that the proper place for diagnostic records is in the individual patients notes or more futuristically in an electronic form or smart card. These records are properly the responsibility of the hospital records department or recipient primary care physicians and if pathologists have reason to doubt the reliability of such systems then it is better to draw the attention of the appropriate authorities to the problem rather than to try and rectify the problem by local duplication and prolonged laboratory storage.

The National Pathology Accreditation Advisory Council in 1987 produced minimum retention periods for various laboratory records and diagnostic materials. In the introduction it comments that 'Much longer retention times may be desired and maintained by individual laboratories and practitioners to meet their particular requirements and by institutions engaged in teaching or research. This applies particularly to histopathology and cytology records for which many authorities see the need for a retention period of at least 50 years'. As the introduction says, this is not without its implications for storage facilities and as long as minimum periods are met then any further period is for local evaluation.

REQUIREMENTS FOR STORAGE AND RETENTION OF DOCUMENTS AND SPECIMENS

The requirements for the storage and retention of documents and specimens are shown in Figure 4.16.

System	Storage and retention of documents and specimens
ISO 9001:1994	**4 Quality system requirements** **4.5 Document and data control** **4.5.1** *General* 'The supplier shall establish and maintain documented procedures to control all documents and data that relate to the requirements of this International Standard.....' *and note 15 says,* ' Documents and data can be in any form of media, such as hard copy or electronic media' **4.16 Control of quality records** The supplier shall establish and maintain documented procedures for identification, collection, indexing, access, filing, storage, maintenance and disposition of quality records'.
EN 45001:1989	**5 Technical competence** **5.4 Working procedures** **5.4.4** *Records* 'The testing laboratory shall maintain a record system .... It shall retain on record all original observations, calculations and derived data, calibration records and the final test report for an appropriate period................'. **5.4.5** *Handling of test samples or items* 'A system for identifying the samples or items to be tested or calibrated shall be applied either through documents or through marking, to ensure that there can be no confusion regarding the identity of the samples or items and the results of the measurements made............'
OECD - GLP	**10 Storage and retention of records and material** **10.1 Storage and retrieval** **(1)** 'Archives should be designed and equipped for the storage and accommodation and secure storage of'.....*and details what should be stored. It requires an index to be available that will* 'facilitate orderly storage and rapid retrieval', and finally specifies that 'Only personnel authorised by management should have access to the archives' **10.2 Retention** **(1)** 'The following should be retained for the period specified by the appropriate authorities......' *and details what should be retained.* 'Samples should be retained only as long as the quality of the preparation permits evaluation' and 'If the test facility or an archiving contracting facility goes out of business and has no legal successor, the archive should be transferred to the archives of the sponsor(s) of the study(s)'.
CAP - LAP	**Standard II Resources and facilities** *the last sentence of the standard reads* 'There shall be appropriate record storage and retrieval'.
CPA(UK)Ltd	**C Facilities and Equipment** **C6** 'There are appropriate and adequate data storage, retrieval and communications facilities' **C9** 'There are adequate storage facilities for specimens, reagents and records'.

Figure 4.16   **Requirements for storage and retention of documents and specimens**

FURTHER READING

Good Laboratory and Clinical Practices - Techniques for the Quality Assurance Professional. Edited by Carson P A and Dent N J, Heinemann Newnes, Oxford, 1990.

Huber L, Good Laboratory Practice and Current Manufacturing Practice, Hewlett Packard, Germany, 1994.

Retention of Laboratory Records and Diagnostic Material. Commonwealth Department of Health, National Pathology Accreditation Advisory Council, 1987.

The Retention and Storage of Pathological Records and Archives. Report of the Working Party of the Royal College of Pathologists, 1995.

Chapter 5

Organisation and Management

INTRODUCTION

It is useful at this point to consider very briefly what we mean by the term *organisation* and the term *management*. To organise something can be defined as 'to form parts or elements of something into a structured whole'*, and an organisation can be described as 'a business or administrative concern united and constructed for a particular purpose'*. Such structures are represented in an *organisation chart* or as it is sometimes called an *organogram*. An organisation chart can be defined as in Figure 5.1. There is no correct way to create an organisation chart, it can be used to show the relationship of different functional units within an organisation, or to show staff accountability or both.

An organisation chart

'.......is a diagram representing the management structure of a company, showing the responsibilities of each department, the relationship of each department to each other, and the hierarchy of management'

The Collins English Dictionary 3rd Edition updated 1994

Figure 5.1   Definition of an organisation chart

The word 'management' is used in organisations in two distinct ways, to describe either 'the members of the executive or administration of an organisation'* or to describe 'the task of management'*. A number of quality and accreditation systems refer to 'management responsibilities'. This term includes both meanings of 'management'. The first word, 'management' meaning 'the members of the executive or administration of an organisation' and the second word 'responsibilities' meaning 'the task to be carried out'. The task of managing has been usefully and simply defined in terms of the nature of a manager's job (Figure 5.2).

There are many different ways in which a pathology laboratory can be organised. In large hospitals, particularly large teaching hospital laboratories, the pathology disciplines operate as separate autonomous departments. In the medium sized district general hospital the pathology laboratory is composed of a group of individual disciplines or departments.

---

*The Collins English Dictionary 3rd Edition updated 1994 ISBN 0 00 470678-1

Each department will normally have one person in overall charge, and these 'heads of department' will be medically qualified pathologists or scientists with the appropriate education and training. These heads of department will form, perhaps with a technical and/or business manager, the management team. One of the heads of department would be elected or appointed to act as chairman or director of the pathology laboratory. In small hospitals or their equivalent, the laboratory is often a single entity with no separate departments.

The manager's job

'......can be broadly defined as 'deciding what should be done and then getting other people to do it'

The first task comprises -
  • setting objectives
  • planning (including decision making)
  • setting up the formal organisation

The second task consists of -
  • motivation
  • communication
  • control (including measurement)
  • the development of people

The Reality of Management - Rosemary Stewart (1986)

Figure 5.2   The nature of a manager's job.

From the point of view of accreditation systems, it is not so much how different laboratories are organised, or what the head of department is called that is important, but that the scope of the laboratory's work and management's responsibilities are clearly defined. However, some accreditation systems, such as CAP-LAP and CPA(UK)Ltd, require that, whatever the structure, there should be pathologists or clinical scientists who are appropriately qualified to take overall responsibility. In other words, management has to be appropriately qualified.

The functioning and effectiveness of a pathology laboratory can be hindered or enhanced by the quality of its relationship with its parent body or host organisation. In most cases this will be a hospital, but in some cases it will be a holding company, and management of the laboratory will be independent of any of the hospitals which it serves. This relationship is a management relationship *outside the laboratory*. Equal in importance, is how the organisational structure and management *within the laboratory* impacts upon the way it functions. The role of heads of department or of the laboratory is pivotal, both in relationship to the management of the parent body and in being effective managers within the laboratory. Some accreditation systems recognise the importance of these distinct types of relationships and require compliance with specific standards.

In this chapter the purpose and content of a quality manual is discussed, and emphasis is placed on how it can set the scene for the way in which a laboratory responds to the standards of a particular quality or accreditation system. It also discusses the role of a head of department/management outwith and within pathology.

HEAD OF DEPARTMENT/MANAGEMENT

In some accreditation systems the requirement for a head of department is explicit and the responsibilities, qualifications and training for such a post clearly defined. In other systems the term 'management' encompasses the same issues as 'head of department' but, although responsibilities are clearly defined, no requirements as to qualifications, training and experience are specified. In this section where the term 'head of department' is used it can be taken as synonymous with 'management' although the responsibilities of a head of department are not confined to a managerial role.

RESPONSIBILITIES OF A HEAD OF DEPARTMENT

The responsibilities of a head of department will be dependent on the type of work a laboratory performs. This in turn dictates the type of accreditation sought. Thus the management's responsibilities in a laboratory seeking GLP accreditation would include, amongst other things, agreeing *study plans* with sponsors, and the designation of an individual with appropriate qualifications, training and experience as the study director of a particular study. These duties are equivalent to discussing what service the doctor requires and who will be the contact person for advice and consultation in a pathology laboratory servicing a district general hospital.

To provide a consultant advisory service supported by adequate scientific diagnostic facilities, in the laboratory, at the bedside, in the outpatient department and in the home, covering all aspects of laboratory investigation including the interpretation of results and advice on further appropriate investigation.

Department of Health HM(70)50 August 1970

Figure 5.3 A definition of hospital laboratory services

A useful definition of 'Hospital Laboratory Services' was published by the Department of Health in 1970 (Figure 5.3). This definition requires that the head of such a service would have both professional (scientific and clinical) and managerial roles. The Audit Commission for Local Authorities and National Health Service in England and Wales, in a report 'The Pathology Services - A Management Review', confirms this by pointing to the complexity of the pathologist/scientist interlinking professional and managerial roles (Figure 5.4).

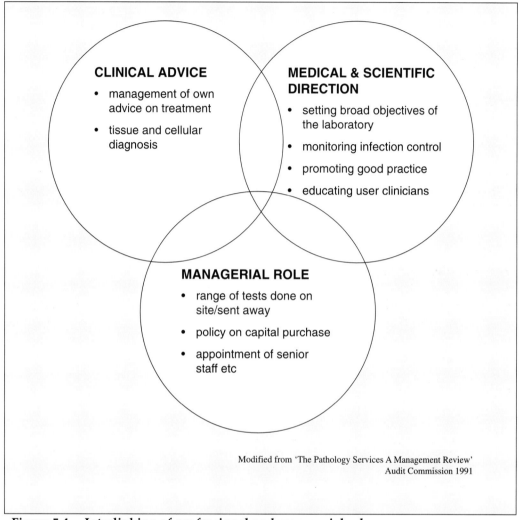

CLINICAL ADVICE
- management of own advice on treatment
- tissue and cellular diagnosis

MEDICAL & SCIENTIFIC DIRECTION
- setting broad objectives of the laboratory
- monitoring infection control
- promoting good practice
- educating user clinicians

MANAGERIAL ROLE
- range of tests done on site/sent away
- policy on capital purchase
- appointment of senior staff etc

Modified from 'The Pathology Services A Management Review'
Audit Commission 1991

Figure 5.4   Interlinking of professional and managerial roles

In the CAP-LAP standards the responsibilities and role of the director are clearly stated (Figure 5.5). Some of these responsibilities can be seen to clearly fall into one of the professional or managerial roles shown in Figure 5.4, but others fall into the interlinking areas.

Section A   Qualifications, responsibilities and role of the director

To function effectively in fulfilling the duties and responsibilities as director of the pathology or medical laboratory service, the director should possess a broad knowledge of clinical medicine, basic medical sciences, clinical laboratory sciences, and operations. The Director should have the appropriate training and background to be able to discharge the following responsibilities:

1. **Medical Significance, Interpretation, and Correlation of Data**
    Make judgements about the medical significance of clinical laboratory data and communicate effectively in interpreting laboratory data and relating correlations to referring physicians.

2. **Anatomic Pathology**
    Perform anatomic pathology procedures as appropriate.

3. **Consultations**
    Provide consultations to physicians regarding the medical significance of laboratory findings as appropriate.

4. **Medical Staff Privileges**
    Serve as an active member of the medical staff as appropriate, for those facilities served.

5. **Interaction with Physicians/Patients/Administrators/Agencies**
    Relate and function effectively with applicable accrediting and regulatory agencies, appropriate administrative officials, the medical community, and the patient population served.

6. **Standards of Performance**
    Define, implement, and monitor standards of performance in quality control, quality assurance, cost-effectiveness of the pathology service, and other ancillary laboratory testing programmes as appropriate.

7. **Monitoring and Correlation of Laboratory Data**
    Monitor all work performed in the laboratory to determine that medically reliable data are being generated; correlate laboratory data for diagnosis and patient management.

8. **Quality Assurance Responsibilities**
    Assure that the laboratory participates in the monitoring and evaluation of the quality and appropriateness of services rendered, within the context of the quality assurance program appropriate for the institution, regardless of testing site(s).

9. **Personnel**
    Ensure that there are sufficient qualified personnel with adequate documented training and experience to supervise and perform the work of the pathology laboratory.

10. **Strategic Planning**
    Perform planning for setting goals and developing and allocating resources appropriate to the medical environment.

11. **Administrative and Management Responsibilities**
    Provide effective and efficient administration of the pathology service including budget planning and control with responsible financial management.

12. **Educational Responsibilities**
    Provide educational direction for the medical and laboratory staff, and participate in educational programs of the institution as appropriate.

13. **Research and Development Responsibilities**
    Plan and direct research and development appropriate to the facility.

14. **Reference Laboratories**
    Select all referral laboratories in accordance with Standard II.

Figure 5.5   CAP-LAP Standard I - Interpretative notes, section A

The responsibilities described form a useful starting point from which to create a job description of a director of the pathology laboratory or for the head of an individual discipline or department.

QUALIFICATIONS OF THE HEAD OF DEPARTMENT

In some accreditation systems there is a specific requirement to have a director or head of department, and this requirement is coupled to the experience and qualifications necessary for the post holder. In CAP-LAP Standard I, section B of the interpretation says that the requirement is for a director of pathology who is 'responsible for the overall operation and administration of the laboratory to assure that quality patient services are delivered' but that 'The director need not perform all responsibilities personally' and can delegate administrative, medical and technical responsibilities to appropriate personnel. Section C says 'When the director cannot adequately discharge all the responsibilities appropriate for the pathology or laboratory service, the services of a qualified consulting pathologist shall be retained.' A consulting pathologist is defined as 'A pathologist who periodically visits the laboratory and serves the role of a consultant, as contrasted with the role of director of laboratories'.

STANDARD I DIRECTOR AND PERSONNEL REQUIREMENTS

The pathology service shall be directed by a physician or doctoral scientist qualified to assume professional, scientific, consultative, organisational, administrative, and educational responsibilities for the service. Generally, it is medically preferable that the director be a board certified pathologist. The director shall have sufficient authority to implement and maintain the Standards.

When a non-pathologist physician or doctoral scientist serves as director, such individual must be qualified by virtue of documented training, expertise, and experience in the areas of analytical testing offered by the laboratory. Where the functions of the laboratory so require, the services of a qualified consulting pathologist shall be retained. In all facilities where anatomic pathology services are provided, a pathologist shall perform such services.

Special function laboratories shall be directed by either a physician who is qualified to assume professional responsibility for the special function laboratory or a qualified doctoral scientist with documented training, expertise, and experience in the appropriate specific clinical discipline and area of testing.

The location, organisation, or ownership of the laboratory shall not alter the requirement of this Standard, its interpretation, or its application.

Figure 5.6   CAP-LAP requirement for a director

The qualifications required for a director are a part of the standard itself (Figure 5.6) and are further defined by Section A Qualifications, responsibilities, and role of the director (Figure 5.5). In this section the director is required to have appropriate training and background to be able to discharge certain responsibilities. In this sense the responsibilities define the experience, education and training required in order to be a director.

The CPA(UK)Ltd Standard B1 (Figure 5.7) differs from the CAP-LAP standard in that it does not prescribe an overall director of pathology but starts at the level of the individual discipline or department within the pathology laboratory, and the guidelines deal with qualifications, experience, education and training required. This is further borne out in Standard A2 which requires that 'There is a documented line of managerial accountability from the head of the applicant (for accreditation) department to senior management in the organisation concerned'. Thus, the responsibility for running the department and therefore for implementation and maintenance of the CPA(UK)Ltd standards lies with the head of department.

B1 Each discipline is professionally directed by a pathologist or clinical scientist of equivalent status

Guidelines:

1. Evidence of training and/or experience in that speciality as normally exemplified either by the MRCPath or its equivalent or by appointment as a consultant or equivalent in that speciality by a properly constituted NHS Appointments Advisory Committee

2. Evidence of continuing practice in that speciality; and

3. Evidence of participation in continuing medical education relevant to that speciality.

4. There must be adequate arrangements for cover during staff absences.

5. There has to be regular on-site involvement

For laboratories without on-site consultants the following points need to be satisfied for each discipline:

    i) A written definition of the sessional input for each consultant sufficient to meet the needs of the service.

    ii) Documented attendance at regular departmental meetings to review service issues and set standards.

    iii) Regular on-site attendance as needed to match the needs of the service; normally at least weekly.

    iv) Interpretative consultant advice should be available readily and within a timescale appropriate to the urgency of the clinical situation.

    v) Clinicians should be aware of the availability of consultant advice and have ready access to it at all times.

Figure 5.7   CPA(UK)Ltd Section B Staffing and direction - Standard B1

The formal qualifications required will differ in individual countries and can form part of a country's legislation (CLIA'88) or be a requirement at interview, see section 1 of the guidelines in Figure 5.7.

REQUIREMENT FOR DESIGNATED RESPONSIBILITIES OF MANAGEMENT / HEAD OF DEPARTMENT

The requirements for designated responsibilities of management or of a head of department in the different quality and accreditation schemes is summarised in Figure 5.8. ISO 9001:1994 and OECD-GLP systems use the term 'management' to encompass the same issues as head of department.

System	Responsibilities of Management / Head of Department
ISO 9001:1994	**4. Quality system requirements** **4.1 Management responsibility** **4.1.1 *Quality policy*** **4.1.2 *Organisation*** *4.1.2.1 Responsibility and authority* *4.1.2.2 Resources* *4.1.2.3 Management representative* **4.1.3 *Management review***
EN 45001:1989	**5. Technical competence** **5.1 Management and organisation** '........A document showing the organisation and distribution of responsibilities of the testing laboratory shall be available and kept up-to-date' *(This paragraph is the nearest to a description of management responsibilities)*

OECD - GLP	**1. Test facility organisation and personnel**
	1.1 Management's responsibilities
	(1) Test facility management should ensure that the Principles of Good Laboratory Practice are complied with in the test facility.
	(2) at a minimum it should:
	   a) Ensure that qualified personnel, appropriate facilities, equipment, and materials are available;
	   b) Maintain a record of the qualifications, training, experience and job description for each professional and technical individual;
	   c) Ensure that personnel clearly understand the functions they are to perform and where necessary, provide training for these functions;
	   d) Ensure that health and safety precautions are applied according to national and/or international regulations;
	   e) Ensure that appropriate Standard Operating Procedures are established and followed;
	   f) Ensure that there is a Quality Assurance Programme with designated personnel;
	   g) Where appropriate, agree to the study plan in conjunction with the sponsor;
	   h) Ensure that amendments to the study plan are agreed upon and documented;
	   i) Maintain copies of all study plans;
	   j) Maintain a historical file of all Standard Operating Procedures;
	   k) For each study ensure that a sufficient number of personnel is available for its timely and proper conduct;

	l) For each study designate an individual with the appropriate qualifications, training, and experience as the Study Director before the study is initiated. If it is necessary to replace a Study Director during a study, this should be documented; m) Ensure that an individual is identified as responsible for the management of the archives.
CAP - LAP	**Standard I Director and personnel requirements** *(see Figures 5.5 and 5.6)*
CPA(UK)Ltd	**A Organisation and management** **A2** 'There is a documented line of managerial accountability from the head of the applicant department to senior management in the organisation concerned' **B Staffing and direction** *(see Figure 5.7)*

Figure 5.8   **Requirements for designated responsibilities of management/head of department**

ISO 9001:1994 is a quality system standard which can be applied to any type of organisation wishing to ensure the quality of its functioning and it is not to be expected that it would use the terms director or head of department.

In OECD-GLP, in the first paragraph headed 'Test facility organisation and personnel', there are three sub sections which detail the responsibilities of Management, the Study Director and Personnel. Everybody who works in the GLP facility is classed as personnel. The responsibilities of management are shown in Figure 5.8. In EN45001:1989, which is concerned only with technical competence of testing laboratories, there is no direct reference to management responsibilities. The requirements of CAP-LAP and CPA(UK)Ltd have been outlined in Figures 5.5, 5.6 and 5.7.

RELATIONSHIP WITH PARENT BODY

The importance to pathology of a good relationship with its parent body or host organisation has been highlighted in the summary of a report prepared by the Audit Commission for Local Authorities and National Health Service (NHS) in England and Wales, 'Critical Path - An Analysis of the Pathology Services'. It says 'At present there is much conflict between laboratory management and general managers who often have only a hazy knowledge of pathology, but who see steadily rising costs against a background of constrained NHS budgets.

They have responded by tightly controlling inputs while laboratory staff for their part face steadily increasing demand. This 'adversarial management' should be replaced by a new relationship, with authority delegated to laboratories, who in return must be able to satisfy general managers that they are managing their resources well. To do this, they need to set up clear lines of authority with effective methods for controlling resources and deploying staff to the best effect - once again firmly based on sound information'

> **A2** There is a documented line of managerial accountability from the head of the applicant department to senior management in the organisation concerned.
>
> **A3** There are formal arrangements for meetings between senior laboratory staff and management or controlling advisory groups to review the service, set objectives and make appropriate financial arrangements.

Figure 5.9 CPA(UK)Ltd Section A Organisation and management - Relationship with parent body

The requirement for a relationship between management and the pathology laboratory in different quality and accreditation systems depends partly on how the word management is interpreted - whether it means being within the laboratory or outwith the laboratory. In the CPA(UK)Ltd system, which has its origins in the laboratory sections of hospital accreditation systems, the standards A2 and A3 in the section entitled 'Organisation and Management' indicate clearly the requirements for a relationship with the parent body or host organisation (Figure 5.9).

RELATIONSHIPS WITHIN THE LABORATORY

The way in which a laboratory is organised and managed will affect not only the quality of the end product but also have a marked affect on the staff who work in the laboratory. Organisations must be structured to meet local needs, and the way in which they are managed should still follow some fundamental principles (Figure 5.10).

> - clear demarcation of responsibilities
> - clear reporting lines
> - well established and well used lines of communication
> - functions discharged at an appropriate level
>
> 'The Pathology Services: A Management Review'
> Audit Commission (1991)

Figure 5.10 Fundamental principles for organisation and management

PROCEDURE FOR THE ORGANISATION AND MANAGEMENT OF PATHOLOGY

The proposed content of a procedure for the organisation and management of pathology is given in Figure 5.11. The scope and purpose of such a procedure is the organisation and

Content of procedure	References to figures in text
1.0 Purpose and Scope	
2.0 Responsibility	
3.0 References	
4.0 Definitions	
5.0 Documentation	
6.0 Action and methods	

6.1 The Pathology Management Boardl
      6.1.1 Chairperson, deputy chairperson and secretary
      6.1.2 Membership and co-option
      6.1.3 Responsibilities of members
	(see page 7/19 of Figure 5.15)

6.2 Sub committees and working groups
      6.2.1 Quality Assurance Unit sub committee
      6.2.2 Health and Safety sub committee
      6.2.3 Working Groups	

6.3 Frequency of meetings
      6.3.1 Pathology Board
      6.3.2 Sub committees
      6.3.3 Working Groups	

6.4 Agenda of meetings
      6.4.1 Attendance
      6.4.2 Minutes of previous meeting
      6.4.3 Financial report
      6.4.4 Reports from sub committees and working
           groups
      6.4.5 Annual Review of Objectives
      6.4.6 Reports from departmental meetings
      6.4.7 Any other business	

6.5 Minutes of meetings
      6.5.1 Format and numbering
      6.5.2 Distribution	

6.6 Communications
      6.6.1 Annual Review of Objectives
      6.6.2 Minutes of the Board
      6.6.3 Senior Staff meetings
	(Figure 6.14)

Figure 5.11   Content of a procedure for the organisation and management of pathology

management of the pathology laboratory and the services it provides, and this would include the preparation of a business plan and an annual review of objectives. In St Elsewhere's Hospital Trust, the Director of Pathology would be responsible for implementation of procedure and the main records would be the minutes of meetings of the Board and its subcommittees and working groups.

The requirements of the different quality and accreditation systems suggest that at least two subcommittees are required to cover quality assurance (see Chapter 11) and health and safety (Chapter 8). The proposed membership has been mentioned in the model quality manual (page 7/19 of Figure 5.15). The chairperson could be the Director of Pathology, or it could rotate between Heads of Department. In addition to defining the membership the responsibilities of individual members should be defined. The Head of Histopathology in this structure would be accountable managerially to the Director of Pathology and would provide the board with information required to ensure the proper functioning of that discipline.

The frequency of meetings and its subcommittees should be defined and will depend on how much of the day to day management is conducted at the Board and how much is delegated to subcommittees or working groups. The balance between what should be dealt with by the board and what should be dealt with by subcommittees and working groups is a difficult one. The board should perhaps be more concerned with strategic rather than operational matters, and membership of subcommittees should be seen as an opportunity for a broader group of staff to participate in the management of pathology. For example the Management Review required in paragraph 4.1 of ISO 9001 could be undertaken by a full meeting of the Board or by a group appointed by the Board. The Board should meet at least once a month if it is going to maintain continuity and effectively communicate its decisions.

The agenda of the Board meetings should have an agreed structure which would include reports from subcommittees and working groups on a regular basis. The minutes should record decisions taken, and where further action is required it should carefully define the responsibility for reporting back and the time limit. The minutes should be numbered in a defined manner, for example, 45/1996 would denote the forty fifth minute of the Board in 1996. The minutes of the Board and its subcommittees should provide a visiting inspector or assessor with the clear impression that the Board is able not only to make decisions but also to implement them within the resources available.

Figure 5.10 suggests some fundamental principles for organisation and management which are covered in the preceding paragraphs of this section. However, it also requires that there are 'well established and well used lines of communication'. This subject is developed under staffing in Chapter 6.

QUALITY MANUAL

In the previous chapter it was indicated that only some accreditation systems require a quality manual (Figure 4.14). However, it is a good idea to develop one as it serves to introduce the scope and purpose of the laboratory and its policies, and to create an organisational structure for documentation. There are a number of texts which give information on the format and content of a quality manual including the document ISO 10013:1995(E) Guidelines for developing quality manuals.

In the Netherlands the Co-ordinating Committee for the promotion of quality control of laboratory research and testing pertaining to the Health Care Sector (CCKL), an umbrella for organisations offering 'Laboratory Care in the Netherlands' used as a basis the ISO 9000 series of standards and EN 45001, to produce standards in a publication called 'Code of Practice for the implementation of a Quality System in the Health Care Sector'(CCKL Code of Practice). Standard 2.1 states that 'The laboratory must have a unified quality system, laid down in a quality manual which pertains to the laboratory's work'. To assist laboratories in the implementation of this standard, the Netherlands Clinical Chemistry Association (NVKC) have also produced a 'Model Quality Manual'(NVKC Model Quality Manual) which is available as hard copy or as a word processing template.

A group of Scandinavian Clinical Chemists have published a paper entitled 'A quality manual for the clinical laboratory including the elements of a quality system'. This paper is currently under consideration by the Board of the Scandinavian Society for Clinical Chemistry (NFKK) for possible adoption as an 'NFKK recommendation'. Several quality and accreditation systems have served as background for this work including ISO 9001, EN 45000, ISO/IEC Guide 25, and papers which led to the formation of CPA(UK)Ltd. For convenience this work is referred to as the NFKK Quality Manual.

PURPOSE OF A QUALITY MANUAL

A quality manual is a useful document in relation to a number of different groups of people (Figure 5.12). The head of department and management have the final responsibility for quality policy in a laboratory and it ensures that they understand the commitments that are being made to quality.

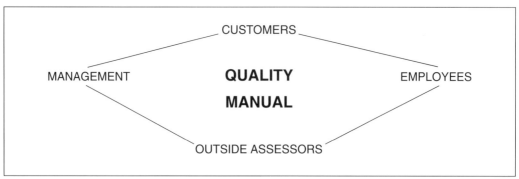

Figure 5.12 Purposes of a quality manual

It provides a document that enables employees to understand management's commitment to a quality policy and use it to focus their activities.

When the time comes for outside assessors to visit the laboratory and assess compliance with the standards of whatever accreditation system is being adopted, the quality manual forms a starting point for the assessment. Finally, it can be given to a customer to assure them of a commitment to quality. In this last sense it can be used in marketing to attract new customers. With these different uses in mind it is important that the quality manual should be up to date, clearly and succinctly written, and attractively produced.

PREPARATION AND CONTROL OF THE QUALITY MANUAL

Once the management decision has been made to document the quality or accreditation system in a quality manual, the job is normally delegated to a Quality Manager/Officer who will work with a Quality Assurance Group to co-ordinate its production. The same process of document control as described in Chapter 4 will apply to the quality manual. Any copies issued outside the pathology laboratory for purposes of information to present or potential customers should be clearly marked as uncontrolled copies. The United Kingdom Accreditation Service produces 'The Quality Manual - guidance for preparation' which recommends that each section be numbered separately, e.g. section 3 would have page 3.1, 3.2 etc. Whilst this makes for ease of revision and updating as only single sections have be replaced, when revised it makes overall control slightly more complex. Further references for general guidance are given in Further Reading.

CONTENT OF THE QUALITY MANUAL

The content of a quality manual as suggested in ISO 10013:1995(E) is shown in Figure 5.13. The opening pages of a quality manual are discussed in the following paragraphs and illustrated in Figure 5.15 which shows the opening seven pages of the Quality Manual for the Pathology Department of St. Elsewhere's Hospital Trust.

TITLE, SCOPE AND FIELD OF APPLICATION

The title page or the cover should give the title, scope and field of application of the quality manual and the usual document control information. If the quality manual is to cover the whole of the pathology laboratory then it should be stated clearly. However if, for example, Histopathology were not to be involved then this should be stated explicitly rather than by default. Continuing the document design developed in Chapter 4, the front page might be as shown in page 1/19 of Figure 5.15. On the second page or inside the front cover there should be a history and circulation page (page 2/19 of Figure 5.15).

TABLE OF CONTENTS

The table of contents should contain the title of the main sections and the numbering of the sections should be shown together with the page number. If the quality manual is based directly upon an International Standard such as ISO 9001:1994 then the contents numbering should follow the numbering in the standard, e.g. 4.1 Management responsibility, 4.2 Quality system, 4.3 Contract review, etc. Page 3/19 of Figure 5.15 shows a contents page which is based upon a number of different guidelines which have interpreted of EN 45001:1989 for pathology laboratories.

---

1. Title, scope and field of application.

2. Table of contents.

3. Introductory pages about the organisation concerned and the manual itself.

4. Quality policy and objectives of the organisation.

5. Description of the organisation, structure, responsibilities and authorities.

6. Description of the elements of the quality system and any references to documented quality system procedures.

7. Definitions section, if appropriate.

8. Index to the quality manual.

9. Appendix for supportive data.

Based on ISO 10013:1995(E) Guidelines for developing quality manuals

---

Figure 5.13   Content of a quality manual

INTRODUCTORY PAGES ABOUT THE ORGANISATION AND THE MANUAL ITSELF

The introductory page of the quality manual should provide basic information about the organisation itself and about the quality manual (Figure 5.15 page 4/19).

THE QUALITY POLICY AND OBJECTIVES OF THE ORGANISATION

After the introductory pages then follows the laboratory's quality policy and objectives. An example of a brief quality policy statement suitable for an individual discipline or a pathology laboratory using the ABC accreditation system is given in Figure 5.14. Quality policies vary greatly in emphasis and a very different quality policy is given in Figure 5.15 page 5/19 which is from the NFKK Quality Manual guidelines.

A DESCRIPTION OF THE ORGANISATION, RESPONSIBILITIES AND AUTHORITIES

This section should contain information concerning the relationship between the pathology laboratory and the parent body or host organisation. If the quality manual is written for an individual pathology discipline, then the relationship of that department to the pathology laboratory and the host organisation should be included (page 6 of Figure 5.15). In a number of accreditation systems there is a clear requirement for this relationship with a parent body. The top level organisation, responsibilities and authorities within the pathology laboratory must be clearly stated. The use of organograms in this section is encouraged. The descriptive text should be brief but should refer to appropriate procedures for detailed explanation (Figure 5.15 page 7/19).

'The Pathology Service shares the corporate objectives of St Elsewhere's Hospital Trust and contributes to their fulfilment by providing a consultative and analytical service which meets the standards laid down by professional and other appropriate bodies, in particular those promulgated by the ABC Accreditation System.

It is recognised that such standards can only be achieved and maintained by adopting an innovative attitude and investment in research and development. Our staff are our most important resource, and personal development through education and training is encouraged.'

Figure 5.14   An example of a quality policy

A DESCRIPTION OF THE ELEMENTS OF THE QUALITY SYSTEM AND ANY REFERENCES TO DOCUMENTED QUALITY SYSTEM PROCEDURES

This section of the quality manual will contain a series of policy statements with regard to the implementation of the provisions, principles, criteria or standards set by the particular quality or accreditation system. These policy statements then indicate the procedures which have been created to implement the particular policy and to comply with the standard. As shown earlier, one purpose of a quality manual is to be able to give it to actual or potential customers and if possible it should be less than twenty five pages.

Ideally a pathology laboratory would have a quality manual for the whole of the laboratory. If each discipline chooses to have its own quality manual it should include the quality policy of the host organisation and of the pathology service as a whole.

St Elsewhere's Hospital Trust	QM 000 001
	Edition 1
PATHOLOGY LABORATORY	Page 1/19

QUALITY MANUAL

This document, together with specified procedure manuals, represents the Quality Policy of the Pathology Laboratory of St Elsewhere's Hospital Trust.

It is compiled to meet the requirements of the ABC Accreditation System and similar national and international standards.

All procedures contained herein are mandatory within the Pathology Laboratory.

EDITION No:	*Edition 1*
OPERATIVE DATE:	*29-May-95*
REVIEW DATE:	*29-May-96*
REPLACES:	*n/a*
LOCATION:	*000 Quality Assurance Unit* *000 Director of Pathology* *100 Biochemistry* *200 Haematology* *300 Microbiology* *400 Histopathology*
AUTHOR: signature: date:	*John Qualimann*
AUTHORISED BY: signature: date:	*Director of Pathology*
COPY No.	*1/6*

MANAGEMENT PROCEDURE

Figure 5.15 Opening pages of a quality manual

St Elsewhere's Hospital Trust	QM 000 001
	Edition 1
PATHOLOGY LABORATORY	Page 2/19

HISTORY PAGE

Edition No	Date	Comment
1	29-May-95	
2		
3		
4		
5		

CIRCULATION LIST

Copy No	Post	Name	Signature
1	000 Quality Manager	John Qualiman	
2	000 Director of Pathology		
3	100 Head of Biochemistry		
4	200 Head of Haematology		
5	300 Head of Microbiology		
6	400 Head of Histopathology		

MANAGEMENT PROCEDURE

Figure 5.15   Opening pages of a quality manual (cont).

St Elsewhere's Hospital Trust	QM 000 001
	Edition 1
PATHOLOGY LABORATORY	Page 3/19

TABLE OF CONTENTS

MANAGEMENT PROCEDURE

Figure 5.15 Opening pages of a quality manual (cont).

St Elsewhere's Hospital Trust	QM 000 001
PATHOLOGY LABORATORY	Edition 1 Page 4/19

0.0 INTRODUCTION

0.1 PATHOLOGY SERVICES

The Pathology Laboratory of St Elsewhere's Hospital Trust is situated in the main hospital building on Level 5 East Wing. It is composed of four departments, Biochemistry, Haematology, Microbiology and Histopathology, and is part of the clinical Directorate of Diagnostic and Therapeutic Services.

St Elsewhere's Hospital Trust provides a wide range of services to the population of St Elsewhere and the surrounding district of East Loanshire. The resident population is approximately 560,000. In addition to the usual facilities of a District General Hospital there are two specialised units, a renal dialysis unit and a cardiac transplant unit, which serve the whole county of Loanshire.

The Pathology Laboratory provides services to the main hospital and to Thorbury Hospital for the severely mentally handicapped. Twice daily courier runs for collection of samples, and electronic transmission of results, enables the provision of effective pathology services for the 350 primary care physicians and their patients in East Loanshire. The Pathology Laboratory is also responsible for the provision of all near patient testing facilities in the main hospital.

The postal address is:-

                Pathology Laboratory,
                St Elsewhere's Hospital Trust,
                Eastside Street,
                ST ELSEWHERE
                East Loanshire,   Telephone   (0800) 100200
                EL7 5XX   FAX   (0800) 300400

Further information on the services provided, and telephone numbers, are provided in the Pathology Services - USERS HANDBOOK, copies of which can be obtained from the Pathology Business Manager telephone 0800 000201

0.2 THE QUALITY MANUAL

The Quality Manager is responsible to the Director of Pathology and with the members of the Quality Assurance Unit is responsible for the creation and control of the Quality Manual. The 'Procedure for document creation and control' [MP 000 001] details the procedures for the formatting, preparation and control of all documentation including the Quality Manual. The Quality Manual together with the Procedure manuals indicated below, form the Quality System of the Pathology Laboratory of St Elsewhere's Hospital Trust.

- Quality procedures manual
- Management procedures manual
- Laboratory procedures manual
- Clinical procedures manual

MANAGEMENT PROCEDURE

Figure 5.15   Opening pages of a quality manual (cont).

St Elsewhere's Hospital Trust	QM 000 001
	Edition 1
PATHOLOGY LABORATORY	Page 5/19

1.0 QUALITY POLICY OF THE LABORATORY

The aim of the Pathology Laboratory of St Elsewhere's Hospital Trust is to provide clinically useful information through the laboratory analysis of samples from patients, taking into account the resources allocated by the Trust. The reported data should be reliable and their uncertainties should be in accordance with the clinical needs and the appropriate technical standards of the profession.

The Quality Policy is implemented by the following means:-

- Proper sample collection, stabilisation, transport, sample preparation and identification;

- Reliable analytical work so that systematic and random errors do not exceed specified limits;

- Turnaround time within specified limits, inter alia for emergency measurements within one hour, and for rare routine measurements within one week after receipt of samples;

- Data reported in a clear form and supplemented with relevant information, including reference intervals, to allow reliable clinical interpretation;

- Appropriate communication with the clinicians so that the results will be interpreted and logically integrated into further (clinical and laboratory) evaluation of the patient, and clinicians become aware of unexpected problems and errors.

MANAGEMENT PROCEDURE

Figure 5.15 Opening pages of a quality manual (cont).

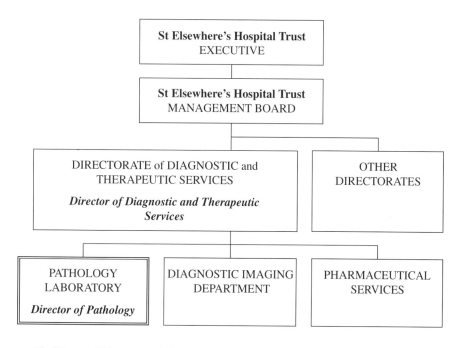

St Elsewhere's Hospital Trust	QM 000 001
	Edition 1
PATHOLOGY LABORATORY	Page 6/19

2.0 A DESCRIPTION OF THE ORGANISATION, RESPONSIBILITIES AND AUTHORITIES

2.1 RELATIONSHIP TO THE HOST ORGANISATION

The Pathology Laboratory is part of the clinical Directorate of Diagnostic and Therapeutic Services. The organisational relationships of that Directorate within St Elsewhere's Hospital Trust are shown below:

```
                    St Elsewhere's Hospital Trust
                           EXECUTIVE

                    St Elsewhere's Hospital Trust
                        MANAGEMENT BOARD

   DIRECTORATE of DIAGNOSTIC and              OTHER
      THERAPEUTIC SERVICES                 DIRECTORATES

  Director of Diagnostic and Therapeutic
              Services

   PATHOLOGY        DIAGNOSTIC IMAGING      PHARMACEUTICAL
   LABORATORY          DEPARTMENT              SERVICES

 Director of Pathology
```

The Director of Diagnostic and Therapeutic Services is a member of the St Elsewhere's Management Board and is represented on the Executive by the Medical Director of the Trust.
The *Director of Pathology* is managerially responsible to the Director of Diagnostic and Therapeutic Services.
The Director of Pathology is the delegated Budget Holder for the Pathology Laboratory within the Directorate of Diagnostic and Therapeutic Services.

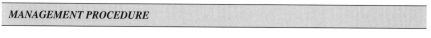

MANAGEMENT PROCEDURE

Figure 5.15   Opening pages of a quality manual (cont).

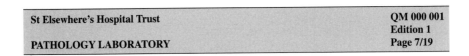

2.2 ORGANISATION AND RESPONSIBILITIES WITHIN THE PATHOLOGY LABORATORY

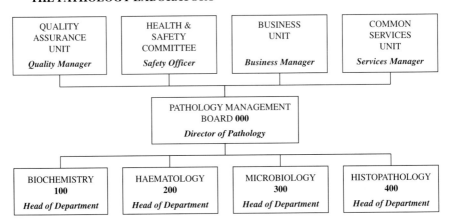

The Pathology Laboratory has four main departments, each with a Head of Department. In departments with more than one Consultant Pathologist or Scientist, the headship is held on a rotating basis. In addition, there are two units and one committee which provide the supporting services for the Pathology Laboratory. Each of these units has a manager or supervisor. The three Managers are responsible directly to the Director. The Safety Officer reports to the Head of Microbiology as a member of the Management Board. The Management Board of the Pathology Laboratory is composed as follows:-

- Director of Pathology
- Heads of Departments
- Quality Manager
- Business Manager
- Common Services Manager

conducted according to the Procedure for the organisation and management of pathology [MP 000 001]. The *Safety Officer* attends the Management Board as required.

The *Quality Manager* is employed half time on Quality Assurance and half time as the Safety Supervisor.

The *Business Manager* is full time and responsible for the laboratory's Business and Computing Systems. The Computer Manager reports to the Business Manager.

The Common Services Manager is full time and responsible for the reception, secretarial and clerical services, for blood collection, for transport and purchasing.

MANAGEMENT PROCEDURE

Figure 5.15   Opening pages of a quality manual (cont).

FURTHER READING

Audit Commission. The Pathology Services - A Management Review. HMSO, London, 1991.

Dybkaer R, Jordal R, Jorgensen P T, et al. A quality manual for the clinical laboratory - including elements of a quality system. Proposed guidelines. Scand J Clin Lab Invest 1993:53 (Suppl 212); 60-77.

ISO 10013:1995(E). Guidelines for developing quality manuals.

Model quality manual. Bureau NVKC, Kredenberg 139A, 3511 BG Utrecht, The Netherlands, 1992.

Munro-Faure L , Munro-Faure M and Bones E. Achieving the New International Quality Standards: A Step-by-Step Guide to BS EN ISO 9000. Pitman Publishing London, 1995.

Stewart R. The Reality of Management. Pan Books Ltd, London, 1986.

The Quality Manual, Guidance for preparation, M16 1996 United Kingdom Accreditation Service, London.

Chapter 6

Staffing

INTRODUCTION

The way in which an organisation attracts, develops, motivates and retains staff determines the quality of the service it provides and whether it is responsive to the changing needs of its customers. It is not surprising therefore to find that quality and accreditation systems contain a number of standards which focus on personnel matters. The previous chapter dealt with certain staffing matters, discussing both the role of management/head of department, and the relationship of the laboratory to its parent body or host organisation.

This chapter is not to be seen as a comprehensive treatise on personnel management but focuses on three areas which are of common concern in quality and accreditation systems and where suitable documentation provides evidence of compliance with standards. Firstly, staffing and administration which includes staff structures and accountability, staff numbers and job evaluation, staff recruitment and selection, job descriptions and personnel records. Secondly, the area of staff development including induction procedures, education, training and staff appraisal, and thirdly, the communication with staff.

STAFFING AND ADMINISTRATION

STAFF STRUCTURE AND ACCOUNTABILITY

In Chapter 5 the concept of organisation charts was discussed. In the model quality manual (page 7 of Figure 5.15) there is an organisational chart for St.Elsewhere's Pathology Laboratory which shows both the structure of the laboratory and the accountability of senior staff to the Director of Pathology. Organisation charts which show staff accountability are sometimes termed accountability charts, but in this text the 'organisation chart' is used to cover both laboratory structure and staff accountability. Such a chart is an essential part of a *job description*, and can be complemented by a written description of staff relationships. Examples of such charts are given in sample job descriptions (Figures 6.5 and 6.6).

STAFF RESOURCES AND JOB EVALUATION

It is always a vexed question in any industry as to how many staff are required to do a particular job, and pathology laboratories are not alone in this. A number of accreditation standards make reference to there being 'sufficient personnel' or 'appropriate staff' but none give a clear indication as to what sufficient or appropriate actually means. This leaves the task of evaluating compliance to such standards as a matter of informed judgement. In practical terms this means that the appropriateness of staffing is evaluated indirectly by whether a quality service is provided.

The nature and number of staff required by a laboratory has to be constantly kept under review as the nature and quantity of the work changes, as new technologies make their impact, and as new organisational structures emerge such as joint Biochemistry/Haematology departments. When a member of staff leaves an organisation it is always a good point at which to evaluate that job and decide whether it is still required in its current form. The annual staff appraisal which is discussed later in this chapter is another opportunity to review an individual's role in relation to the needs of the organisation.

STAFF RECRUITMENT AND SELECTION

Often the first contact that a potential employee has with an organisation will be through responding to an advertisement in a newspaper or professional journal. The laboratory may also have open days for the general public, co-operate with local schools in arranging work experience for senior pupils, or participate in careers conventions. These contacts are important, particularly in attracting locally recruited staff.

Advertisements should have an attractive format and contain a clear indication on how to obtain further information and who to contact to make an appointment for an informal visit. The information sent to a potential applicant should include a job description, a person specification, information about the laboratory and its host organisation, and a job application form.

The role, format, and content of the job description is discussed below but it is worth mentioning at this stage that once a job has been defined, the next task is to create a profile of a person who would be suitable for the post. This profile is often called a *person specification* and there are a number of different ways in which it can be constructed. Figure 6.1 shows a person specification form for a personal secretary to the head of the Haematology department of St Elsewhere's Hospital Trust, based upon the Munro - Fraser system.*

---

*Recruitment and Selection, Advisory Booklet No.6, 1983; ACAS 1983

	St Elsewhere's Hospital Trust	MF 000 014

St Elsewhere's Hospital Trust | MF 000 014
PATHOLOGY | Edition 1
Page 1/1

PERSON SPECIFICATION FORM

    1. JOB TITLE   *Departmental Secretary*

    2. LOCATION   *Haematology Department*

    3. JOB NUMBER   *MF 2JD 005*

	Essential	**Desirable**
IMPACT ON OTHER PEOPLE	*Acceptable bearing and speech*	*Pleasant manner, bearing and speech.*
QUALIFICATIONS AND EXPERIENCE	*'O' level English language or equivalent. Ability to audiotype accurately, and to operate office machines. Experience of general office work.*	*'O' level maths or equivalent. RSA III typing. Experience of using simple statistical information. Experience of staff supervision.*
INNATE ABILITIES	*Quick to grasp a point*	*Ability to assess priorities and make decisions.*
MOTIVATION	*Personal identification with service given by the department. Interest in efficiency of administration*	
ADJUSTMENT	*Steady, self-reliant, good at making friendly relationships with colleagues at all levels.*	*Able to cope with stress and pressure from different user departments.*

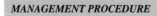

MANAGEMENT PROCEDURE

Figure 6.1   **A completed person specification form**

THE JOB DESCRIPTION - ITS ROLE

From what has already been said regarding job descriptions it is clear that they play a pivotal role in organisational management. Figure 6.2 indicates some of the most important functions of a job description.

Job evaluation	• Essential to the process of job evaluation
Staff selection, recruitment, and induction	• Gives the potential applicant a view of the nature of the job
	• Provides a common understanding of the content of the job between the job applicant and manager/employer
	• Enables job holder and manager to define the position of the job in the organisational structure
Staff appraisal and training	• Provides a basis on which to set objectives for the job holder and manager
	• Helps in the appraisal of both job and personal performance
	• Enables the identification of education and training needs of job holder

Figure 6.2   Functions of a job description

A job description has been defined as 'A detailed written account, agreed between management and worker, of all the duties and responsibilities which together make up a particular job'.* Job descriptions should be prepared for all members of the pathology laboratory including the heads of departments.

---

*The Collins English Dictionary 3rd Edition updated 1994   ISBN 0 00 470678-1

Job descriptions should be seen as separate from a *person specification* and the *terms and conditions of employment*. An example of a person specification has been given in Figure 6.1. Job descriptions are often produced which contain terms and conditions of employment and, although it is a matter of choice as to whether the job description should contain such items, job descriptions are best kept as clear and straightforward as possible. Typical items for terms and conditions of employment are shown in Figure 6.3.

- The employer's name.
- The employee's name.
- The date employment began.
- The job title.
- The amount of pay and the interval between payments.
- Hours of work.
- Holiday pay and entitlement.
- Sick pay arrangements.
- Pension arrangements.
- Notice periods for termination of employment.
- Grievance and appeal arrangements.
- Disciplinary rules

Figure 6.3   Terms and conditions of employment

THE JOB DESCRIPTION - FORMAT AND CONTENT
It is important that the format of job descriptions is the same throughout the laboratory and that similar jobs have similar content if they occur in different parts of the same laboratory. For example, if laboratory assistants are employed in different disciplines within pathology then, although the job descriptions in each situation might vary in the detailed content, they should reflect the same levels of responsibility. If a number of different people are writing job descriptions it is important to give one individual the task of checking for format and style.

The job description should normally contain the items shown in Figure 6.4. The *job title* should be easily understood throughout an organisation and not contain any element of sex discrimination, for example the job title 'laboratory cleaner' should be used rather than 'cleaning lady'. The *location* states where in the pathology laboratory the individual is employed.

The *reference number* of a job description is a reference to the job and not to the individual employed in that job. It can either use the eight digit codes shown in the 'Procedure for documentation preparation and control' (Figure 4.13) or have a separate numbering system. By slightly modifying the system given in the 'Procedure for documentation preparation and control', **MF 0JD 005** might be the code for the Pathology Computer Manager (**MF** = **M**anagement **F**orm, **0** = Pathology, **JD** = **J**ob **D**escription, **005** = Job Description for a Pathology Computer Manager). Some posts, such as that of Pathology Computer Manager, will require separate and distinctive job descriptions, but at the level of Medical Laboratory Assistant (Haematology) the same job description could be used for the three posts at that level in that department (see Figure 6.6).

- **Job title**

- **Location** within the organisation, i.e. department or section

- **Job reference**/Job number

- **Organisation chart** or diagram

- **Main purpose of the job** in the form of a brief statement

- A list of **Main duties and responsibilities**

- **Joint review and the job description**

Figure 6.4   The content of a job description

Not many job descriptions include an *organisation chart* but it is probably the most satisfactory way of conveying to an individual employee their position in an organisation and to whom they are accountable. Two different examples are given in Figures 6.5 and 6.6 which are model job descriptions for a Pathology Computer Manager (job reference number, MF 0JD 005) and a Medical Laboratory Assistant (job reference number, MF 2JD 011) respectively.

The *main purpose of the job* should be brief and concise and aim to convey to the reader the main aspects of the job. The *main duties and responsibilities* can be subdivided into different areas if that makes the presentation easier to follow. The focus should be on what the job holder does rather than on how they do it. Each phrase should start with an action verb in the third person singular, present tense, such as assist, analyse, prepare, perform, report etc. The paragraph, *joint review and the job description* introduces the idea that the review is a shared activity between the manager and the employee and that at an annual joint review the content of a job might change.

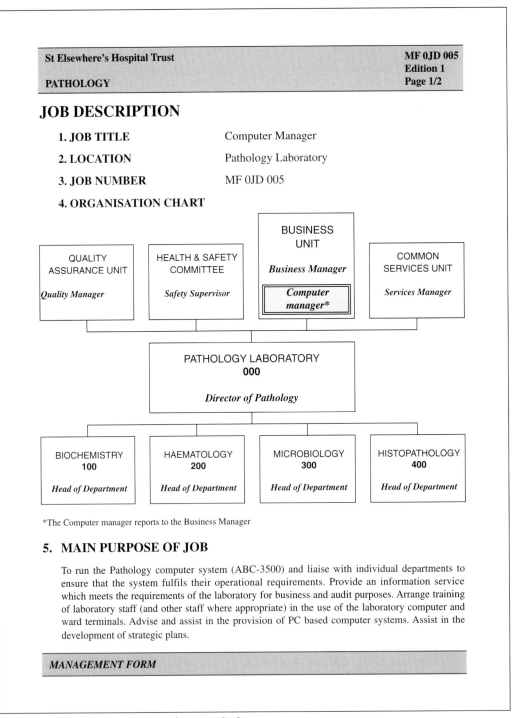

Figure 6.5   Job description for a pathology computer manager

St Elsewhere's Hospital Trust	MF 0JD 005
	Edition 1
PATHOLOGY	Page 2/2

6. MAIN DUTIES AND RESPONSIBILITIES

6.1 PATHOLOGY COMPUTER SYSTEM (ABC-3500)
- Implement and maintain the procedure for management of the laboratory computer.
- Maintain the computer hardware and software, including peripherals and communications, by ensuring maintenance contracts are in place.
- Ensure appropriate hardware and software upgrades are undertaken and records kept.
- Maintain the computer hardware and software register (including personal computers).
- Maintain and manage the database.
- Ensure adequate and secure backup and data storage.
- Produce and update procedures for ABC users and provide ongoing training programmes.

6.2 INFORMATION SERVICE
- Produce invoices for Pathology customers.
- Provide monthly statements of workload and income and expenditure, by department and cost centre.
- Support Clinical Audit activities by the production of data sets.

6.3 PERSONAL COMPUTER (PC) SYSTEMS
- Provide hardware support for PC systems.
- Arrange for software training and support for current word-processing, spreadsheet, database and presentation packages.
- Arrange for software training and support for current costing package.

6.4 STRATEGIC PLANNING
- Provide advice on all future developments in computing and liaise with the Hospital Information Technology Manager.

6.5 GENERAL RESPONSIBILITIES
- Comply at all times with the Laboratory Safety Policy.
- Report/ensure that any defect which may affect safety at work is brought to the attention of the designated supervisor.
- Respect information obtained in the course of duties performed and refrain from disclosing such information without the consent of the employee/patient, or person entitled to act on their behalf, except where disclosure is required by law or by the order of a Court, or is necessary in the public interest.

7. JOB DESCRIPTION AND JOINT REVIEW

The Job Description reflects the present requirement of the post. The job description will be reviewed, in consultation with the job holder, as and when duties and responsibilities change. Such reviews will normally take place at the annual joint review meeting.

Prepared by	Date ....
Job holder's signature	Date ....
Manager's signature	Date ....

MANAGEMENT FORM

Figure 6.5   Job description for a pathology computer manager (cont).

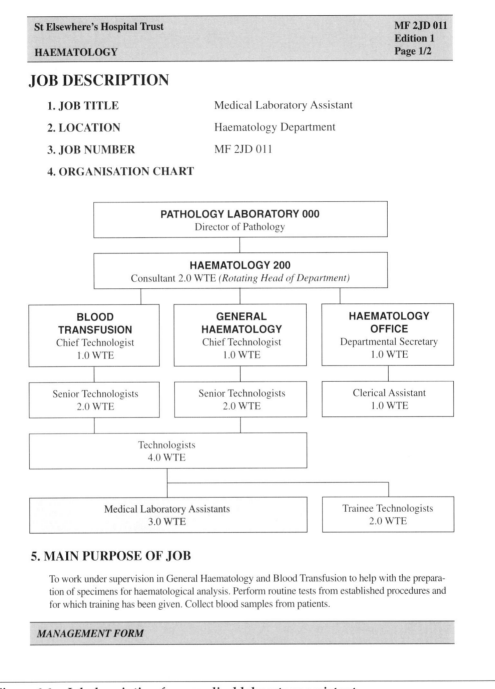

St Elsewhere's Hospital Trust	MF 2JD 011
	Edition 1
HAEMATOLOGY	Page 1/2

JOB DESCRIPTION

1. JOB TITLE   Medical Laboratory Assistant

2. LOCATION   Haematology Department

3. JOB NUMBER   MF 2JD 011

4. ORGANISATION CHART

PATHOLOGY LABORATORY 000
Director of Pathology

HAEMATOLOGY 200
Consultant 2.0 WTE *(Rotating Head of Department)*

BLOOD TRANSFUSION	**GENERAL HAEMATOLOGY**	**HAEMATOLOGY OFFICE**
Chief Technologist 1.0 WTE	Chief Technologist 1.0 WTE	Departmental Secretary 1.0 WTE
Senior Technologists 2.0 WTE	Senior Technologists 2.0 WTE	Clerical Assistant 1.0 WTE

Technologists
4.0 WTE

Medical Laboratory Assistants 3.0 WTE	Trainee Technologists 2.0 WTE

5. MAIN PURPOSE OF JOB

To work under supervision in General Haematology and Blood Transfusion to help with the preparation of specimens for haematological analysis. Perform routine tests from established procedures and for which training has been given. Collect blood samples from patients.

MANAGEMENT FORM

Figure 6.6   Job description for a medical laboratory assistant

6. MAIN DUTIES AND RESPONSIBILITIES

All duties will be performed according to written laboratory procedures and after appropriate training by a designated supervisor.

6.1 SPECIMEN COLLECTION, REGISTRATION AND PREPARATION

- Perform venepuncture on patients.
- Sort and identify specimens received.
- Register patient details and tests required on the laboratory computer.
- Prepare samples where appropriate for analysis.

6.2 TECHNICAL DUTIES

- Perform certain tests under supervision and keep records of test results.
- After checking by designated supervisor, enter test results on laboratory computer.
- Use and operate equipment such as centrifuges, automated equipment, pipettes and computer terminals.

6.3 GENERAL DUTIES

- Prepare solutions and reagents.
- Clean and sterilise laboratory equipment, shelves, bench tops and sinks.
- Dispose of contaminated material including sharps.
- Undertake any other responsibility which may be reasonably allocated by designated supervisor

6.4 GENERAL RESPONSIBILITIES

- Comply at all times with the Laboratory Safety Policy
- Report/ensure that any defect which may affect safety at work is brought to the attention of the designated supervisor.
- Respect information obtained in the course of duties performed, and refrain from disclosing such information without the consent of the employee/patient, or person entitled to act on their behalf, except where disclosure is required by law or by the order of a Court, or is necessary in the public interest.

7. JOB DESCRIPTION AND JOINT REVIEW

The Job Description reflects the present requirement of the post. The job description will be reviewed and revised, in consultation with the job holder, as and when duties and responsibilities change. Such reviews will normally take place at the annual joint review meeting.

Prepared by...	Date...
Job holder's signature...	Date...
Manager's signature	Date...

MANAGEMENT FORM

Figure 6.6   Job description for a medical laboratory assistant (cont).

PERSONNEL RECORDS

Personnel records are an important part of any organisation. If the organisation is large then it is likely to have a personnel department which will either keep staff records within the department or at least require that records in the pathology laboratory are kept to a certain standard and format. In OECD-GLP the main components of staff or personnel records are three fold, a record of formal qualifications (sometimes called a curriculum vitae), the job description, and the record of training and experience. Good practice in personnel management suggests fuller records should be kept and the items required are indicated in Figure 6.7.

Personal details	• name/sex/date of birth/address • education/qualifications • tax code/insurance number • next of kin • name, address and telephone number of doctor • details of any disability
Employment details	• record of posts held with dates, job titles and salary progression
Job description	• copy of current job description
Terms and conditions of employment	*(see Figure 6.3 for further information)*
Staff induction checklist	*(see Figure 6.9 for further information)*
Training record	• date and details of internal and external courses and conferences attended
Staff appraisal records	*(see Figure 6.13 for further information)*
Occupational health record (may be held in occupational health department)	• immunisations • eyesight checks etc.
Absence record	• sickness • lateness (authorised/unauthorised)
Accident record	
Record of disciplinary action	

Figure 6.7   The personnel record

REQUIREMENTS FOR STAFFING AND ADMINISTRATION

The requirements of different accreditation systems in relation to staff and administration are shown in Figure 6.8.

System	Staffing and Administration
ISO 9001:1994	**4. Quality system requirements** **4.1 Management responsibility** **4.1.2 *Organisation*** *4.1.2.1 Responsibility and authority* 'The responsibility, authority and the interrelation of the personnel who manage, perform, and verify work affecting quality shall be defined and documented........' *4.1.2.2 Resources* 'The supplier shall identify resource requirements and provide adequate resources, including the assignment of trained personnel.........'
EN 45001:1989	**5. Technical competence** **5.1 Management and organisation** '........The testing laboratory shall be organised in such a way that each member of personnel shall be aware of both the extent and limitation of his area of responsibility.....' '........A document showing the organisation and distribution of responsibilities of the testing laboratory shall be available and kept up-to-date' **5.2 Personnel** 'The testing laboratory shall have sufficient personnel.........for their assigned function' '.......Information on the relevant qualifications, training and experience of the technical personnel shall be maintained by the laboratory'
OECD - GLP	**1. Test facility organisation and personnel** **1.1 Management's responsibilities** **(2)** at a minimum it should: (a) Ensure that qualified personnel..............are available (b) Maintain a record of qualifications, training, experience and job description for each professional and technical individual.
CAP - LAP	**Standard I Director and personnel requirements** **D Personnel** 'There shall be sufficient number of qualified laboratory technologists, technicians and other laboratory staff to perform the required tests promptly and proficiently.......'. '.........The laboratory shall maintain documentation of the technical personnel authorised to perform procedures.........'
CPA(UK)Ltd	**Staffing and direction** **B2** There are appropriate numbers of staff with the required training to ensure a satisfactory operation of service. **B3.** There is a documented line of accountability for all staff. **B4.** The duties and responsibilities of all staff are specified in job descriptions. **B5.** All staff have a contract of employment which clearly states terms and conditions of service.

Figure 6.8   Requirements for staffing and administration

STAFF DEVELOPMENT

INDUCTION

Staff induction is included in this section because it is the first opportunity to orientate a new employee to the work place, and in that sense is the earliest part of staff development. The induction begins during recruitment and selection, but this section will focus from the first day at work onwards. What is important to any new employee, particularly to a school leaver who may have had no previous experience of the work place, is what to do on the first day, where and when to report, who to report to, what to bring, and if arriving by car or bicycle where to park. To block the parking space reserved for the Director of Pathology would not be the ideal way to begin a new job!

The nature of the induction, who does it and when, will vary depending on the size and nature of the laboratory's host organisation; it should however be done in a systematic way and according to a written procedure. As the induction proceeds a record should be kept using a *staff induction checklist*, and the whole process constantly monitored to ensure that all important aspects have been dealt with. This induction checklist should be part of the employees personnel record and provides evidence at an accreditation inspection that an induction scheme is in operation.

The amount of information which needs to be imparted to the new employee may well seem alarming and confusing and should therefore be imparted over a period of time; not too much being attempted on the first day. A number of people will be involved in the induction process, and who does what could be part of the staff induction checklist. If the new employee is coming as a trainee technologist in the Haematology Department, then they might meet the Head of Department briefly and be conducted through the day by the Chief Technologist or an assigned deputy. Some organisations assign a suitable person of similar grade to befriend the new recruit in the first few weeks, showing them where the toilets are, where to eat lunch, and inviting them to join in some social activity like a visit to a bowling alley one evening.

St Elsewhere's Hospital Trust has a personnel department which holds induction courses only every two months and therefore a large amount of the initial work has to be done by pathology laboratory staff.

Whatever the format of the induction checklist it is important that the process imparts to new employees information categorised under headings shown in Figure 6.9.

Organisational information

- nature of the organisation, its history and where the employee's department fits.
  (information given in the model Quality Manual (Figure 5.15) would be suitable)

Procedural information

- terms and conditions of employment *(see Figure 6.3 for further information)*

- disciplinary and grievance procedures

- health and safety procedures

- fire and bomb procedures

- standards or codes of dress

- rules on entering and leaving the premises

Job information

- a job description including an organisation chart *(see Figures 6.5 and 6.6)*

- details of any training

- procedures for obtaining equipment, stationery, or tools

Personal information

- how salaries are paid

- location of dining room

- location of changing facilities and toilets

Team information

- information about the employees immediate workplace

- informal information to make the individual feel part of the team

Figure 6.9   Categories of information for new employees

TRAINING

In different countries there are different arrangements for training staff but the content of the training will also depend upon the level of entry of the staff, and their role in the organisation. Some new employees will come to their post fully qualified having undertaken their education and training in other organisations, but for some it will be their first job. For the former a familiarisation programme at induction may be all that is required, but for the new entrant a documented training scheme will be very important. In many professions, postgraduate training is undertaken only in institutions which are accredited for training purposes. The professional bodies which represent these professions will have a system of monitoring the institutions providing the training and will provide training log books as well as visiting the trainees at regular intervals to ensure that they are being provided with the appropriate opportunities to gain experience and training.

Functions common to two or more pathology specialities

1. Purpose and relationships of the clinical laboratory
2. Safe working procedures in the laboratory
3. Sterilisation and disinfection procedures
4. Waste disposal, including that of specimen remains
5. Phlebotomy
6. Reception, sorting and labelling of specimens
7. Input to and maintenance of laboratory computer system: derivation of work sheets for qualified staff
8. Separation of blood serum and plasma
9. Manual transcription and recording of laboratory data
10. Cataloguing and storage of specimens
11. Weighing and measuring, making up solutions
12. Maintaining working stocks of reagents and consumable items
13. Receiving requests for information by telephone and responding appropriately

Competencies required in particular pathology specialities

14. Clinical Chemistry (Chemical Pathology)
15. Clinical Cytogenetics
16. Clinical Immunology
17. Clinical Microbiology
18. Diagnostic Virology
19. Haematology Laboratory
20. Hospital transfusion Laboratory
21. Histopathology and Cytopathology

Manual for Training and Competence Assessment of Medical Laboratory Assistants
Second Edition 1992 Department of Health (UK)

Figure 6.10 Medical laboratory assistant activities

In the United Kingdom there is a grade of laboratory worker called a Medical Laboratory Assistant (MLA) whose instruction and training is entirely on the job (see Figure 6.6 for job description). The Department of Health published a Manual for training and competence assessment of MLA's. Figure 6.10 indicates the range of training and competencies required. The first section deals with MLA work common to two or more specialities and the second section with competencies needed in particular pathology disciplines. The first two common competencies are obligatory items and any grouping of functions or parts of functions can then be used for a particular MLA post.

The initial part of any training programme may have content which overlaps with the content of an induction programme, particularly in areas of familiarisation with the organisation and department, and aspects of health and safety. The important thing is that if there is overlap which can be useful in reinforcing a message, then the material used is the same for both induction and training.

CONTINUING EDUCATION

There is always a need for continuing education and training in an organisation such as a Pathology Laboratory. The form it will take depends on the needs of the individual and of the bodies which increasingly regulate the continuing accreditation of individuals. Monitoring the need for continuing education can usefully take place at the annual joint review. It is important that all staff have ready access to library and information services and a quiet place in which to study. Resources must be available to allow staff to attend appropriate meetings.

APPRAISAL

A number of accreditation systems require that the organisation should have some form of documented 'staff appraisal' scheme. The concept appears under a number of different titles such as employee appraisal, performance review, annual review, etc. and staff appraisal in some organisations is linked to schemes of remuneration. The type of staff appraisal which is adopted by an organisation will depend on the staff to be appraised and on the way in which the organisation conducts its business. A useful definition to set the scene for the purpose of staff appraisal in the context of laboratory accreditation is given in Figure 6.11.

Staff appraisals...

'....regularly record an assessment of an employee's performance, potential and development needs. The appraisal is an opportunity to take an overall view of work content, loads and volume, to look back on what has been achieved during the reporting period and agree objectives for the next'.

ACAS Advisory booklet No.11.
Employee appraisal

Figure 6.11   Definition of staff appraisal

Staff appraisal is not only a 'once a year' formal activity but in a well run organisation is supplemented by frequent informal contact between the immediate supervisor and the staff member. A word of praise or a timely piece of cautionary advice is just as valuable as the formal appraisal.

There are a number of different approaches to staff appraisal. Some schemes rely on grading qualities or skills, such as honesty and communication, rating them on a scale from unacceptable to excellent. Other schemes involve assessing against objectives or targets and result in a written assessment of the job holder by the manager. Further Reading at the end of this chapter gives a number of useful references. No one scheme is ideal but what is important is that the benefits of staff appraisal shown in Figure 6.12 are realised by all parties.

Benefits to the job holder

- Opportunity to discuss all aspects of the job, with the boss, in depth and away from pressures of daily work load.
- Clarifies how to contribute to the objectives of the department, and the aims of the organisation.
- Identifies strengths and weaknesses, building on the former and addressing the latter.
- Gives clear direction as to what is expected in the job, involving the holder in planning their work and their future.
- Recording the interview and action plan signifies a mutual commitment.

Benefits to the boss

- Creates an opportunity for managers to think seriously about what they expect of their staff and clarifies plans for the future.
- Opportunity to recognise new ideas and tackle problem areas.
- Clarifies and improves relationships between the two parties, and strengthens the role of the manager as a leader.

Benefits to the organisation

- Appraisal represents a visible commitment by an organisation to the importance of its staff.
- Creates opportunity for greater individual effectiveness and commitment to corporate aims.

Modified from Lawson I 'Appraisal and appraisal interviewing'
The Industrial Society (1989)

Figure 6.12   Benefits of staff appraisal schemes

The approach to staff appraisal used at one time by OXFAM has been adapted in Figure 6.13 and sets out a proposed methodology. It includes the necessary forms for an annual or if felt appropriate, more frequent appraisal. This approach to staff appraisal is termed 'Joint review' and this title is important in that it indicates the co-operative nature of the exercise.

St Elsewhere's Hospital Trust	MF 000 013
	Edition 1
PATHOLOGY	Page 1/4

ANNUAL JOINT REVIEW

STAFF MEMBER

To: Name: ....

Job Title: ....

Department: ....

Copy to: Name: ....

Job Title: ....

Department: ....

The purpose of this Review is to enable you and your immediate manager to take stock of how things are going for you at work - in your overall job and specific work plans, in your working relationships with other people, and any other aspects of working with Pathology. In short, Joint Reviews - taking place throughout the Hospital Trust - are designed to promote and sustain good, productive working relationships all round.

Most jobs and people are developing all the time. It is therefore likely that out of the Review will emerge some points for action - by you, your manager, and/or others - to help you and your work develop further during the next year.

The attached papers are provided to help you and your manager obtain maximum benefit from the Review. Topics have been laid out to provide some talking points - but this should not prevent discussion about other aspects of your working life. Please prepare for the Review by going through the papers. If space is insufficient please use additional sheets of paper, numbering them accordingly. A set of these papers is also being sent to your manager who will prepare thoughts for your Joint Review.

As a result of your Review the 'Action Notes' should be completed together with, on the reverse side, any other agreed points which emerge from the discussion. These notes are for your benefit as well as your manager and will be available to your manager's manager if required.

The other working papers will remain in the possession of you and your manager unless you both wish and agree otherwise.

If you have any queries at all about the Joint Review, do please get in touch with the Personnel Department.

MANAGEMENT FORM

Figure 6.13   Joint review form

St Elsewhere's Hospital Trust   MF 000 013
Edition 1
PATHOLOGY   Page 2/4

PREPARATION FOR JOINT REVIEW

1.   **The job**

a)   What are the main tasks or responsibilities in your job?
(Please refer to the job description and note any significant changes over the last year.)

b)   Which areas of your work do you think have gone particularly well during the past year?
(Please say why you think this is.)

c)   Which areas of your work have proved most difficult during the past year?
(Please say why you think this is.)

d)   How would you anticipate your job could develop or otherwise change over the next year?
(Please note any items which you feel should be given priority attention.)

2.   **Working relationships**

a)   Who are your main work contacts?
Please indicate where other people most directly affect, or are affected by, the way you perform your job.

i)   The ones who most directly affect the way I perform my job are:

ii)   The ones who are most affected by the way I perform my job are:

b)   What support and assistance with work do you receive from and give to others?
(Please note instances where this works particularly well or less well.)

i)   Support and assistance received from others:

ii)   Support and assistance given to others:

c)   How would you like to see your working relationships change or develop over the next year?

MANAGEMENT FORM

Figure 6.13 Joint review form (cont).

St Elsewhere's Hospital Trust	MF 000 013
	Edition 1
PATHOLOGY	**Page 3/4**

3. The Department and You

a)   How do you feel in more general terms about working in your department? (Please indicate anything you feel particularly happy or unhappy about in your department and its work.)

b)   How do you see your future within your department? (Please indicate any particular aspirations and ambitions you have.)

4. Other aspects

Are there any other points you would like to raise that have not been covered so far? (Please attach additional sheets as required.)

5. Ideas for Action (joint and individual)

a)   What would you like to see done to help with things indicated above (in Sections 1-4)?

b)   What could you do to help things along?

MANAGEMENT FORM

Figure 6.13 Joint review form (cont).

St Elsewhere's Hospital Trust	MF 000 013
	Edition 1
PATHOLOGY	Page 4/4

ANNUAL JOINT REVIEW

ACTION NOTES

This is a summary of action agreed by:

(Name)..

and their manager

(Name)..

as a result of their discussions on:

(date) ....

Topic	Agreed Action/Training	Whose Action, by when

MANAGEMENT FORM

Figure 6.13 Joint review form (cont).

STAFF COMMUNICATION

MEETINGS

Figure 6.14 shows page 10 taken from the procedure for personnel management [MP 000 003] in St.Elsewhere's Hospital Trust. It shows in diagrammatic form the meetings which take place at different levels in the organisation and the information that passes up and down the system. The direct line of reporting would be from Departmental Management Meetings to the Pathology Management Board, and from Pathology Management to the Board of Directors of the host organisation. These meetings are conducted in a formal manner and minutes made which record the decisions taken and designate who shall take action when it is required. Information regarding the procedure for the organisation and management of pathology, including conduct of the Pathology Management Board and other meetings in pathology, was given in Chapter 5. The Departmental Management Meetings can be conducted in a similar manner. The Senior Staff meetings in Pathology and the Staff meetings in individual departments are less formal and either notes or minutes are taken. These meetings are a very important opportunity for a wider group of staff to participate in the functioning of the laboratory, and for management to learn at first hand the concerns of the staff.

INFORMATION SHARING

Information sharing needs an understanding of what information should be shared and the mechanisms for sharing. In any organisation there is always an informal 'grapevine' through which information or misinformation will travel. In the case of misinformation this can often cause unnecessary distress and concern. If systems are in place for information sharing then the information passing through the system must be reliable and clearly presented. Figure 6.14 indicates information and mechanisms which can be used. The Management Board should produce an annual report and this could include a section on future objectives which would enable employees to gain a better understanding of the organisation and give the pathology laboratory and its departments an indication of how they might organise their own objectives. Briefing notes, produced at regular intervals and either sent to selected individuals for onward dissemination or displayed prominently throughout the organisation, will assist in the process of communication. However, information should not just come down through an organisation but should also travel upwards, either through the medium of minutes of meetings, through feedback during verbal briefings, or other methods such as non-conformance reports in quality systems or through monitoring complaints.

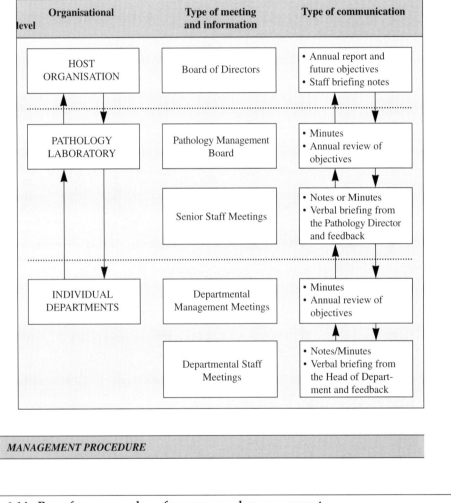

St Elsewhere's Hospital Trust — MP 000 003 Edition 1
PATHOLOGY — Page 10/11

6.7 MEETINGS AND COMMUNICATION

The figure below shows in diagrammatic form the meetings which take place at different levels in the organisation and the type of information that passes up and down the system. The direct line of reporting would be from the Departmental Management Meetings to the Pathology Management Board, and from the Pathology Management to the Board of Directors of the host organisation. These meetings are conducted in a formal manner and minutes are made which record the decisions taken and designate who will take action when action is required.

Organisational level	Type of meeting and information	Type of communication
HOST ORGANISATION	Board of Directors	• Annual report and future objectives • Staff briefing notes
PATHOLOGY LABORATORY	Pathology Management Board	• Minutes • Annual review of objectives
	Senior Staff Meetings	• Notes or Minutes • Verbal briefing from the Pathology Director and feedback
INDIVIDUAL DEPARTMENTS	Departmental Management Meetings	• Minutes • Annual review of objectives
	Departmental Staff Meetings	• Notes/Minutes • Verbal briefing from the Head of Department and feedback

MANAGEMENT PROCEDURE

Figure 6.14 Page from procedure for personnel management

System	Staff development and communication
ISO 9001:1994	**4. Quality system requirements** **4.18 Training** 'The supplier shall establish and maintain documented procedures for identifying training needs and provide for the training of all personnel performing activities affecting quality. Personnel performing specific assigned tasks shall be qualified on the basis of appropriate education, training and/or experience as required. Appropriate records of training shall be kept.'
EN 45001:1989	**5. Technical competence** **5.2 Personnel** 'The testing laboratory shall have sufficient personnel, having the necessary education, training, technical knowledge and experience for their assigned function'. 'The testing laboratory shall ensure that the training of its personnel is kept up-to-date.......'
OECD - GLP	**1. Test facility organisation and personnel** **1.1 Management's responsibilities** '**(2)** at a minimum it should: (c) ensure that personnel clearly understand the functions they are to perform and, where necessary, provide training for these functions.'
CAP - LAP	**Standard I Director and personnel requirements** **D Personnel** 'The director shall ensure that procedures and tests performed by the technical staff are within the scope of education, training, and experience of the individual(s)......' '......The laboratory shall maintain documentation of the qualifications of technical personnel authorised to perform procedures.' 'Provision shall be made for all personnel, including physicians and supervisors, to further their knowledge and skills through on-the-job training, in-service education programs, or attendance at workshops, institutes, and/or professional meetings. In-service education programs shall be provided at defined intervals appropriate for the size and needs of the technical staff. The program content and personnel participation shall be documented.' 'An orientation program shall be provided for each new laboratory employee, and the employee's participation shall be documented.'
CPA(UK)Ltd	**B Staffing and direction** **B6.** Regular staff meetings are held to review services. **B7.** All new staff are given a comprehensive orientation and induction programme, including health and safety **E Staff development and education** **E1.** There is a written programme of training for all trainee members of staff. **E2.** There are appropriately sited facilities available to support training and continuing education. **E3.** There are resources for staff to attend appropriate seminars, meetings and conferences. **E4.** There is a continuing education programme for all staff. **E5.** There is a staff appraisal system.

Figure 6.15 Requirements for staff development and training

REQUIREMENT FOR STAFF DEVELOPMENT AND COMMUNICATION

The references to the requirement for staff development and communication in the different quality and accreditation systems are tabulated in Figure 6.15. It can be seen that training in particular is a major requirement in all systems.

PROCEDURE FOR PERSONNEL MANAGEMENT

The extent to which the Pathology Laboratory has its own procedures for personnel management and the extent to which they are determined by the parent body or host organisation was discussed in the introduction to this chapter. The content of a model procedure is shown in Figure 6.16. It covers a full range of activities, some of which will be provided by the laboratory and some by the parent body or host organisation, and refers to other figures in this chapter for further information.

Content of procedure	References to other figures in the text
1.0 Purpose and Scope	
2.0 Responsibility	
3.0 References	
4.0 Definitions	
5.0 Documentation	
6.0 Action and methods	
6.1 Recruitment and selection	*(Figure 6.1 Person specification form)*
	(Figure 6.3 Terms and conditions of employment)
	(Figure 6.4 Content of a job description)
	(Figures 6.5/6.6 Job descriptions)
6.2 Personnel records	*(Figure 6.7 The personnel record)*
6.3 Induction	*(Figure 6.9 Categories of information for new employees)*
6.4 Training	*(Figure 6.10 Medical Laboratory Assistant activities)*
6.5 Continuing education	
6.6 Joint review	*(Figure 6.13 Joint review form)*
6.7 Meetings and communication	*(Figure 6.14 Page from procedure for personnel management)*
6.8 Disciplinary action	

Figure 6.16 Content of procedure for personnel management

FURTHER READING

Employee appraisal - Advisory Booklet Number 11, 1992; Advisory, Conciliation and Arbitration Service (ACAS).

Employing people - The ACAS Handbook for Small Firms, 1992; ACAS.

Good Laboratory and Clinical Practices ed.Carson PA. and Dent NJ. Heineman Newnes, 1990. Chapter 14 Staff records

Induction of New Employees - Advisory Booklet Number 7, 1992; ACAS.

Lawson I. Notes for Managers - Appraisal and appraisal interviewing, 1989; Industrial Society Press, London.

Manual for Training and Competence Assessment of Medical Laboratory Assistants, 1992; Department of Health (UK) Second Edition.

OXFAM Annual Joint Review of staff (personal communication).

Personnel Records - Advisory Booklet Number 3, 1992; ACAS.

Recruitment and Selection - Advisory Booklet Number 6, 1983; ACAS.

Twine A. Notes for Managers - Job descriptions, 1990; Industrial Society Press, London.

Watts-Davies R. Notes for Managers - Induction, 1990; Industrial Society Press.

Chapter 7

Facilities and equipment

INTRODUCTION

The term 'facilities' is in common use in many quality and accreditation systems and can be defined as 'the means or equipment facilitating the performance of an action* '. In the context of a laboratory, facilities can be interpreted as meaning the premises and services to those premises such as heating, ventilation, computer links, etc., and the equipment or apparatus in those premises. The term 'premises' is defined as 'a piece of land together with its buildings, especially considered as a place of business' and is often described as a 'workplace'. As facilities are closely interrelated to health and safety, the introduction to this chapter will serve in part as an introduction to Chapter 8.

Different quality and accreditation systems may place different emphasis on require-ments for facilities, premises and equipment, and on the health, safety and welfare of staff. However, irrespective of these requirements, individual countries generally have legislation (regulations, codes of practice and guidelines), which set standards for the workplace whether it is a factory, an office block or a pathology laboratory. To illustrate these legislative approaches reference is made in this chapter to the principles which underlie Directives promulgated within the European Community (EC) . These principles not only establish the standards required but also represent a practical approach to the management of premises and equipment, and to ensuring the health, safety and welfare of all persons likely to be affected by the functioning of a pathology laboratory.

The EC currently comprises fifteen Member States and since its beginnings in the Coal and Steel Community (Treaty of Paris, 1951) and the Economic Community and Atomic Energy Community (Treaties of Rome, 1957) it has been concerned with the area of workers' safety. In the EC the implementation of the articles of a treaty is accomplished by a number of dif-ferent legislative processes amongst which is the promulgation of directives (see Figure 7.1). Directives have a particular type of role and although it is binding as to the result to be achieved, it leaves individual Member States the choice of form and methods.

---

*The Collins English Dictionary 3rd Edition updated 1994 ISBN 0 00 470678-1

Article 189

In order to carry out their task and in accordance with the provisions of this Treaty, the European Parliament acting jointly with the Council, the Council and the Commission shall make regulations and issue directives, take decisions, make recommendations or deliver opinions.

A regulation shall have general application. It shall be binding in its entirety and directly applicable in all Member States.

A directive shall be binding, as to the result to be achieved, upon each Member State to which it is addressed, but shall leave to the national authorities the choice of form and methods.

A decision shall be binding in its entirety upon those to whom it is addressed. Recommendations and opinions shall have no binding force.

Note: As amended by Article G(60) of the Treaty on European Union.

Figure 7.1   Article 189 of the Treaty establishing the European Community

In the Single European Act of 1987 there are two articles which relate to Health and Safety. Article 100a requires harmonisation of national legislation and seeks the removal of barriers to trade which are based on different national safety standards. Article 118a, requires the harmonisation of existing Health and Safety laws throughout the European Community (Figure 7.2). Both articles contribute to the improvement of the working

Article 118a

1. Member States shall pay particular attention to encouraging improvements, especially in the working environment, as regards the health and safety of workers, and shall set as their objective the harmonisation of conditions in this area, while maintaining the improvements made.

2. In order to help achieve the objective laid down in the first paragraph, the Council, acting in accordance with the procedure referred to in Article 189c and after consulting the Economic and Social Committee, shall adopt by means of directives, minimum requirements for gradual implementation, having regard to the conditions and technical rules obtaining in each of the Member States.[1]

   Such directives shall avoid imposing administrative, financial and legal constraints in a way which would hold back the creation and development of small and medium-sized undertakings.

3. The provisions adopted pursuant to this Article shall not prevent any Member State from maintaining or introducing more stringent measures for the protection of working conditions compatible with this Treaty.

Note: [1]First subparagraph as amended by Article G(33) of the Treaty on European Union.

Figure 7.2   Article 118a of the Treaty establishing the European Community

environment as well as equal or better protection for workers in the Member States. When Article 118a of the Treaty was added by the Single European Act (1986) the Community's authority in these areas was greatly enhanced. In 1987 the European Commission (which is the executive body of the EC) adopted a comprehensive programme on the safety, hygiene and health at the place of work.* At the same time it set up a system for mutual interchange of information on matters affecting the health and safety of workers at their place of work (OJ L183 of 14.07.1988).

In 1989, Directive 89/391/EEC introduced measures to encourage improvements in the safety and health of workers at work (OJ L183 of 29.06.1989). The directive had a general provision that the employer bears the duty to ensure the safety and health of workers in every aspect related to the workplace. The main principles introduced in this directive are

- The employer must ensure that an assessment is made of the risks to the health and safety at work.

- The employer must ensure that the workers of the undertaking receive information on among other things: the safety and health risks, preventive measures, first aid, fire fighting, the risk assessment.

- The employer must consult workers and/or their representatives on matters concerning their safety and health.

- The employer must ensure that each worker receives adequate and job-specific safety and health training.

- Each worker has an obligation to take care of his/her own safety and health and to make correct use of machinery, dangerous substances, personal protective equipment, etc.

adapted from William Hunter,
Social Europe 3/93 Europe for safety and health at work

Figure 7.3   Main principles of the 'framework directive'

show in Figure 7.3. Article (16) 1 of this 'framework directive' required that following its introduction further individual directives must be adopted and reference will be made to them at appropriate points during this and the following chapters.

In the previous chapter the importance to an organisation of well motivated staff was emphasised. The environment in which staff work and the equipment with which they perform their allocated duties makes a major contribution to their well-being. This chapter looks at the issues raised in different accreditation systems in relation to the premises and equipment used in those premises, and its proper maintenance, calibration and control. Computers will be regarded as equipment in general management terms but further

*(OJ C28 of 03.02.1988) [OJ = Official Journal of the European Communities]

information will be found regarding their functional management in Chapter 9. Responsibilities to the environment outside the workplace is mentioned briefly in this chapter, and health, safety and welfare in the workplace is dealt with in Chapter 8.

PREMISES

The nature and extent of the premises which constitute the pathology laboratory in a hospital are determined by three main factors.

- By the services which are offered by the laboratory, e.g. are clinics or phlebotomy services provided within the laboratory area? Are blood products available on a 24 hour basis from the laboratory?

- The tests offered by the laboratory, e.g. do they use radioisotopes or are pathogenic organisms isolated and cultured?

- and are staff facilities such as rest rooms or seminar/library facilities available within the laboratory area?

With respect to staff facilities it may be that they are provided outside the laboratory itself, in which case ease of access is an important consideration. Also of importance are those areas in a hospital other than the main laboratory where pathology testing is conducted. The management of these 'Near-Patient' or 'Point of Care Testing' facilities is dealt with in Chapter 10.

All samples received by the laboratory for analysis are potentially infective, and a major focus in laboratory management must be the safety and prevention of infection for all laboratory staff and for persons who have a legitimate reason to enter the laboratory. The separation of areas engaged in 'clean' functions, such as staff rest rooms, offices, clinic rooms, mortuary viewing room, from those engaged in 'dirty' activities such as the main laboratories, washing up and autoclaving facilities, post mortem rooms and mortuary facilities is of major importance.

When looking at the requirements in the different quality and accreditation systems three issues are addressed in connection with premises (and their internal environment). The first two issues concern whether or not the premises are appropriate for the services offered and for the functioning of equipment. The third issue is whether the premises and the equipment therein provide a safe and healthy working environment for the staff and for any other persons who may have cause to enter the premises, such as patients or service engineers. Depending on their scope and purpose, pathology laboratories will have a selection of facilities and activities as shown in Figure 7.4. In some cases there will be an overlap between types of facilities, for example a haematologist sometimes sees a patient in their own office in which case it should meet both the requirement as a patient facility and as a haematologist's office. The mortuary and post mortem facilities can sometimes be quite separate from the pathology laboratory but for the purpose of this text they are included.

Facilities	Activities
Patient facilities	• Patient reception • Consultation • Phlebotomy • Sample collection other than blood • Dynamic function tests • Mortuary viewing room
Staff facilities	• Education and training • Welfare
Laboratory and office	• Office work (individual and general) • Specimen reception and handling • Routine analytical work • Research and development • Infection control • Storage of reagents, control material and samples • Storage of consumables • Storage of records • Waste disposal
Special facilities	• Blood banking • Preparation of products for *in vivo* patient administration use (e.g. radioisotopes). • Autoclaving • Mortuary and post-mortem room

Figure 7.4   **Laboratory facilities and activities**

PATIENT FACILITIES

If patient facilities are available within the pathology laboratory then they need to be clearly separated from the laboratories. The requirements for patient facilities are well described in the guidelines to Standard C4 from CPA(UK)Ltd (Figure 7.5). An addition to 'instructions to visitors' might be the provision of instructions appropriate to the area served by the laboratory. In 1992 the UK Government introduced 'The Patients Charter' and hospitals have to demonstrate their degree of compliance with set standards. Such information can provide a further useful guide to items of importance in relation to patients' facilities in a pathology laboratory. For example, there is a standard which reads 'that all health services should make provision so that proper personal consideration is shown to you, for example by ensuring that your privacy, dignity and religious and cul-tural beliefs are respected. Practical arrangements should include meals to suit all dietary requirements, and private rooms for confidential discussions with relatives'.

C4 Where applicable there are adequate facilities for patients.

Guidelines:

1. There should be waiting/reception areas separate from the laboratory which have suitable access, with facilities provided for the disabled. Instructions to visitors should be seen and readable (e.g. by the poorly sighted).

2. Patient WC and hand-washing facilities should be separate from those used by laboratory staff.

3. There should be an examination or phlebotomy room which affords appropriate privacy and recovery facilities.

4. There should be adequate provision for the proper storage of consumables for phlebotomy etc.

5. There should be written policies for specimen collection/dynamic function tests.

Figure 7.5   CPA(UK)Ltd Section C   Facilities and equipment - Standard C4

STAFF FACILITIES

There are two aspects to standards for the provision of staff facilities, firstly those facilities associated with welfare, and secondly those associated with education and training which have been dealt with in Chapter 6. EC Directive 89/654/EEC* concerns 'the minimum safety and health requirements for the workplace', and is the first individual directive resulting from the 'framework directive'.

It has been implemented in the UK as the Workplace (Health, Safety and Welfare) Regulations 1992. With respect to the welfare of staff, the regulations require the provision of sanitary conveniences and washing facilities, drinking water, accommodation for clothing, facilities for changing, and facilities for rest and to eat meals. Of particular interest in relation to staff welfare in laboratories are the standards in relation to the 'accommodation for clothing and facilities for changing' and the 'facilities for rest and to eat meals' (Figure 7.6).

---

*OJL 393, 30.12.1989

Accommodation for clothing and facilities for changing

- Adequate, suitable and secure space should be provided to store workers' own clothing and special clothing. As far as is reasonably practicable the facilities should allow for drying clothing.

- Changing facilities should also be provided for workers who change into special work clothing. The facilities should be readily accessible from workrooms and washing and eating facilities and should ensure the privacy of the user.

Facilities for rest and to eat meals

- Suitable and sufficient, readily accessible, rest facilities should be provided. Rest areas or rooms should be large enough, and have sufficient seats with backrests and tables, for the number of workers likely to use them at any time. They should include suitable facilities to eat meals where meals are regularly eaten in the workplace and the food would otherwise be likely to become contaminated.

- Seats should be provided for workers to use during breaks. These should be in a place where personal protective equipment need not be worn. Work areas can be counted as rest areas and as eating facilities, provided they are adequately clean and there is a suitable surface on which to place food. Where provided, eating facilities should include a facility for preparing or obtaining a hot drink. Where hot food cannot be obtained in, or reasonably near to, the workplace, workers may need to be provided with a means for heating their own food.

- Canteens or restaurants may be used as rest facilities provided there is no obligation to purchase food.

- Suitable rest facilities should be provided for pregnant women and nursing mothers. They should be near to sanitary facilities and, where necessary, include the facility to lie down.

- Rest areas and rest rooms away from the workstation should include suitable arrangements to protect non-smokers from discomfort caused by tobacco smoke.

from Workplace - Health, Safety and Welfare A short guide for Managers
Health and Safety Executive (1994)

Figure 7.6   Staff accommodation requirements

LABORATORY AND OFFICE SPACE

EC Directive 89/654/EEC* which was mentioned in relation to facilities for staff welfare has other requirements which concern general aspects of health and safety in relation to premises. A summary from Workplace - Health, Safety and Welfare, A short guide for Managers, Health and Safety Executive (1994) is shown in Figure 7.7. Nearly all of these requirements relate to physical aspects of the premises, and some are important not only to the health and safety of staff, but also to the proper functioning of equipment or test systems.

---

*OJL 393, 30.12.1989

Mention is made in a number of quality and accreditation schemes to the requirement for long term storage of records, samples and processed material such as slide preparations of different tissues (including blood smears), and to proper storage of disposables, reagents, calibration and quality control material. The failure to provide adequate storage facilities can create significant safety hazards such as blocked evacuation routes.

Safety

- Maintenance

- Floor and traffic routes

- Falls and falling objects

- Transparent or translucent doors, gates or walls and windows

- Openable windows and the ability to clean them safely

- Doors and gates

- Escalators and moving walkways

Health

- Ventilation

- Temperature in indoor workplaces

- Lighting

- Cleanliness and waste materials

- Room dimensions and space

- Workstations and seating

from Workplace - Health, Safety and Welfare; A short guide for Managers, Health and Safety Executive (1994)

Figure 7.7   Physical aspects of premises in relation to health and safety

SPECIAL FACILITIES

The CPA(UK) Ltd system has 44 standards, 41 of which are common to all disciplines in pathology. Of the three discipline-specific standards, one relating to responsibility for infection control (Standard D14) is detailed in Figure 2.15. The remaining discipline specific standards relate to mortuary and post mortem (autopsy) facilities (Standard C2), and to facilities for the storage of blood and blood products (Standard C10). Some information regarding these topics is given in the following paragraphs.

MORTUARY AND POST MORTEM FACILITIES

In the CAP-LAP inspection checklist for Anatomic Pathology and Cytology, the section entitled Autopsy Pathology details some of the key issues concerning mortuary and post mortem facilities. Similar information is given in the guidelines from standard C2 CPA(UK)Ltd and the NPAAC Laboratory Assessment Checklist on Anatomic Pathology. Figure 7.8 gives a list of requirements based on this information.

1. There is sufficient space with adequate separation of 'clean' and 'dirty' areas.

2. The location should be convenient in relation to other pathology and institutional services.

3. Access to the mortuary and post mortem facilities should be controlled.

4. There should be air conditioning and adequate ventilation to eliminate noxious fumes and biological odours.

5. There should be satisfactory lighting.

6. There should be satisfactory provision for refrigerated storage of bodies.

7. There should be satisfactory working arrangements.

8. The autopsy room should be clean and well maintained.

9. A scale or balance should be provided for weighing organs.

10. The range of instruments should be adequate and they should be clean, sharp and well maintained.

11. There should be provision for dictation or recording of findings.

12. There should be conveniently placed photographic facilities available.

13. There should be a locker room and shower available for personal cleanup.

14. There should be appropriate materials available for collection of specimens for special studies (e.g. toxicological, microbiological etc.).

Figure 7.8   Requirements for mortuary and post mortem facilities

STORAGE OF BLOOD AND BLOOD PRODUCTS

Another special situation in pathology concerns the facilities for the storage of blood and blood products. Section 3, 'Preservation of blood and blood products' of the NPAAC Laboratory Assessment Checklist states 'Specific policies regarding temperature control should be established and understood by all personnel. The major concern is the preservation of blood. If there is a power failure or refrigeration failure, arrangements must be made for urgent service and, if necessary, for alternative storage of blood'. The questions which relate to the facilities rather than to procedures used in the management of the facilities are shown in Figure 7.9.

3.1 Cold Storage

    3.1.6 Does each refrigerator in which blood is stored meet the standards recommended by the National Blood Transfusion Committee

    3.1.7 Is the refrigeration space adequate for the needs of the facility

    3.1.9 Is emergency power available for each refrigerator in which blood is stored

    3.1.11 Is deep freeze storage available

    3.1.12 Is liquid nitrogen available

3.2 Temperature recorder

    3.2.1 Is a temperature recorder attached to each refrigerator in which blood is stored

    3.2.3 Is the temperature sensor placed in 150-250 ml of fluid

    NOTE: The location of the sensors (in liquid or air) is controversial. It is recommended that the sensor for the recording system be placed in liquid to reflect the status of stored blood, and the sensor for the visual and audible alarm be left in air to provide an early warning system

3.3 Blood Bank Alarm

    3.3.1 Is there a visual alarm system

    3.3.2 Is there an audible alarm system

    3.3.3 Is the alarm system monitored 24 hours a day (either in the laboratory or away from the laboratory)

    3.3.5 Are the alarms adjusted to be triggered outside the range 2°-8° C

    3.3.6 Does the alarm system function independently of the mains electricity supply

from NPAAC Laboratory Assessment Checklist. Blood banking, blood grouping and cross matching 1981

Figure 7.9   NPAAC requirements for blood and blood products storage facilities

EXTERNAL ENVIRONMENTAL EFFECT OF AN ORGANISATION

In the previous section requirements for the environment within the workplace were discussed, but in this section a broader definition is required. In the UK, BS 7750:1994 Specification for Environmental management systems, defines the environment as 'The surroundings and conditions in which an organisation operates, including living systems (human and other) therein. As the environmental effects of the organisation may reach all parts of the world, the environment in this context extends from the workplace to the global system'. The discovery of specific radioactive isotopes in sheep on the Welsh hills which relates to the emissions caused by the Chernobyl disaster are a graphic reminder of the environment as a global system. One aspect pertinent to the pathology laboratory is the requirement to have procedures for waste management, and this is included in the contents of the Laboratory Health and Safety Handbook (Figure 8.3) in the next chapter. The ISO standard, ISO 14001, on environmental management is due to be published at the end of 1996.

It is important that either the pathology laboratory or its parent body should develop procedures to manage resources efficiently and to minimise detrimental effects they may have on the external environment. In many countries in the world there will be legislation regarding such matters as the disposal of hazardous waste, and the control of emissions into the atmosphere.

---

1. Assessment, control, and reduction of the impact of the activity concerned on the various sections of the environment

2. Energy management, savings and choice

3. Raw materials management, savings, choice and transportation; water management and savings

4. Waste avoidance, recycling, reuse, transportation and disposal

5. Evaluation, control and reduction of noise within and outside the site

6. Selection of new production processes and changes to production process

7. Product planning (design, packaging, transportation, use and disposal).

8. Environmental performance and practices of contractors, subcontractors and suppliers

9. Prevention and limitation of environmental accidents

10. Contingency procedures in cases of environmental accidents

11. Staff information and training on environmental issues

12. External information on environmental issues

modified from Annex I Council Regulations (EEC) No. 1836/93 (1993)

Figure 7.10 Issues to be addressed in developing an environmental policy

Annex I of EC-Council Regulation (EEC), No. 1836/93 of 29 June 1993* which allows voluntary participation by companies in the industrial sector in a Community eco-management and audit scheme, a list of issues to be covered is given (Figure 7.10), all of which have to a greater or lesser extent application to a pathology laboratory.

---

*OJL168/1-18 10th July 1993

REQUIREMENT FOR PREMISES (AND ENVIRONMENT)

The requirements for premises including the internal environment in the different quality and accreditation schemes are shown in Figure 7.11.

System	Premises (and Environment)
ISO 9001:1994	**4. Quality system requirements** **4.1 Management responsibility** **4.1.2** *Organisation* **4.1.2.2** *Resources* 'The supplier shall identify resource requirements and provide adequate resources ...' **4.11 Control of inspection, measuring and test equipment** **4.11.2** *Control procedure* ....g) Ensure that the environmental conditions are suitable for the calibrations, inspections, measurements and tests being carried out . . . . .; **4.15 Handling, storage, packaging, preservation and delivery** **4.15.3** *Storage* 'The supplier shall use designated storage areas or stock rooms to prevent damage or deterioration of product, pending use or delivery. . . . .'
EN 45001:1989	**5. Technical competence** **5.3 Premises and Equipment** **5.3.2** *Premises and environment* The environment in which the tests are undertaken shall not invalidate the test results or adversely affect the required accuracy of measurement........ The testing premises shall be protected as required from excessive conditions such as heat, dust, moisture, steam, noise, vibration and electromagnetic disturbance or interference, and shall be maintained accordingly. They shall be sufficiently spacious to limit the risk of damage or danger and to allow operators to make practical and precise movements.
OECD - GLP	**3. Facilities** **3.1 General** **(1)** The test facility should be of suitable size, construction and location to meet the requirements of the study and minimise disturbances that would interfere with the validity of the study. **(2)** The design of the test facility should provide an adequate degree of separation for proper conduct of each study. *(further detailed requirements are given for the test facility etc.)*
CAP - LAP	**Standard II Resources and Facilities** 'The pathology services shall have sufficient and appropriate space, . . . for the performance of the volume of work . . . ' under the interpretative notes it says, 'The scope of the responsibilities and activities of the pathology service must be delineated. Once this determination has been made, sufficient and appropriate space and equipment must be provided' 'The environment in the laboratory shall be conducive to effective performance of personnel and equipment'

CPA(UK)Ltd	C Facilities and Equipment
	C1 There is appropriate office and laboratory space
	C2 There are adequate mortuary and post-mortem facilities (histopathology only)
	C3 There are suitably located staff facilities
	C4 Where applicable there are adequate facilities for patients
	C5 There is appropriate space available for specimen reception, dispatch and handling
	C8 There is adequate and safe provision of lighting, heating, ventilation, power, gases, water and drainage
	C11 There is a safe environment in accordance with current legislation

Figure 7.11 Requirements for premises (and environment)

EQUIPMENT

Pathology laboratories have a great diversity of equipment, ranging from test tubes to large multichannel analysers and sophisticated staining machines. In the different quality and accreditation systems, three distinct aspects are emphasised to a greater or lesser extent (Figure 7.12). Whether appropriate equipment is provided will be judged in relation to the type, workload and purpose of the work undertaken by the laboratory. Simply stated, a blood glucose meter would not be appropriate for a large laboratory but might be appropriate in a doctor's office. Aspects of the management of equipment and its control and calibration are discussed below.

- Provision of appropriate equipment for the task

- Management of equipment, including written procedures and records for maintenance and records of times it was in use

- Procedures or working instructions for the operation of equipment including records of control and calibration with special reference to measurement uncertainty

Figure 7.12 Key issues for equipment

EQUIPMENT MANAGEMENT

In order that a laboratory continues to have appropriate equipment it is necessary to have a management procedure which includes a continuing assessment of need, and mechanisms for evaluation and purchase. The purpose of equipment management is to ensure that equipment available fulfils the requirements given in Figure 7.13.

This is not the place to give a detailed account of equipment management. This discussion focuses on the records and sources of information which can be called upon to provide evidence that a procedure is being followed properly. With all equipment a file should be maintained which records the assessment and justification of need ('the business case'), the process of selection and the acceptance procedure.

Equipment management ensures that...

- it is suitable for its intended purpose.

- its operation is understood by its users.

- it is in a safe and proper operating condition.

- it meets safety and quality standards and requirements.

- it is stored or operated in appropriate and controlled conditions.

- it satisfies (a) to (d) above in a cost-effective manner.

Adapted from Health Equipment Information No.98 (1991)
Management of Medical Equipment and devices

Figure 7.13 Purposes of equipment management

The selection of equipment involves defining the functional requirements, identifying equipment which would potentially meet those requirements, and ensuring that the equipment meets appropriate safety specifications. A satisfactory level of service support needs to be available and adequate training and documentation (including a user manual) must be provided. Finally, all the revenue consequences need to be identified in order that a cost-effective solution is found. An acceptance procedure needs to be agreed with the manufacturer before an order is finally placed in order that any disputes over fitness for purpose can be resolved against a background of objective specification.

The record of training to operate the equipment should be found in the training records of individual members of staff and the level of competence or responsibility required will be defined in the laboratory procedures or working instructions for using the particular analyser, and in the laboratory procedures for carrying out a particular analysis.

EQUIPMENT INVENTORY

The establishment and maintenance of an equipment inventory should be the starting point for any documentation and records concerning a particular piece of equipment. The purpose of an equipment inventory is to provide information for a number of purposes (Figure 7.14).

Uses of an equipment inventory are to......

- be able to audit whether a piece of equipment was used at a particular time to carry out a particular procedure.

- keep a record of maintenance contracts and servicing.

- assist in replacement planning.

Figure 7.14   Uses of an equipment inventory

Figure 7.15 shows the information required in an equipment inventory database. This unique inventory number for each piece of equipment can be cross-referenced to other documents, such as the procedures/work instructions, which describe how to use the equipment. If the equipment inventory is to be used for replacement planning then additional information regarding the purchase price and projected length of life and replacement costs will need to be included.

An inventory record should include...

- a unique identifier.

- the equipment description and name.

- the manufacturer's name and type identification and serial number.

- date received.

- date placed in service.

- date removed from service

- location in laboratory or hospital.

- condition when received (e.g. new, used, reconditioned).

- maintenance record.

- history of any damage, malfunction, modification or repair.

Figure 7.15   Information required in an equipment inventory

MAINTENANCE AND SERVICING

Whether or not the equipment inventory is held in a computer database or as hard copy, details of the maintenance contract and records of service visits, scheduled or unscheduled, are best kept as a separate computer file or on a separate record sheet. In the case of large complex pieces of equipment requiring frequent user servicing as well as scheduled and unscheduled maintenance, an alternative to keeping such information in the equipment inventory may be a log book for each piece of equipment.

The record of maintenance or servicing should include when it was done, what was done, who did the work, and any record of testing/calibration/acceptance before being put back in use. Some documents required by the laboratory can end up in the accounts department, but copies should be retained in the laboratory. If a backup instrument is used during the servicing, it is important to establish that the two instruments give comparable results. Such a log book may also be the chosen place in which to record calibration data, quality control and reagent changes. The best arrangement will have to be determined for each situation, but always remembering the main objective which is to be able to determine that on a certain day an assay was performed on a particular piece of equipment, a calibration record is available, and the batches of control material and reagents are known.

Before equipment is repaired or serviced on site or at the manufacturers, agent's or elsewhere it is important that, if appropriate, it should be decontaminated by suitably trained staff. Some manufacturers or suppliers require a 'Declaration of contamination status and authorisation to work' before the engineer will commence work. The appropriate form for the pathology laboratory of St Elsewhere's Hospital Trust is shown in Figure 7.16 and is a form required by the procedure for equipment management (Figure 7.17).

St Elsewhere's Hospital Trust	MF 000 043
	Edition 1
PATHOLOGY	Page 1/1

EQUIPMENT SERVICING

DECLARATION OF CONTAMINATION STATUS AND AUTHORISATION TO WORK

TYPE OF EQUIPMENT

INVENTORY NUMBER

TICK WHERE APPROPRIATE

A) This equipment/item has not been used in an invasive procedure or been in contact with blood, other body fluids or pathological samples. It has been cleaned in preparation for inspection, servicing or repair. ☐

B) This equipment/item has been cleaned and decontaminated. The method of decontamination was:- ☐

C) This equipment/item has not been decontaminated. The nature of the risk and the safety precautions to be adopted are:- ☐

I declare that I have taken all reasonable steps to ensure the accuracy of the above information.

Authorised signature....................................... Name (printed)..

Position.. Hospital and Department ....

Tel/Bleep No.. Date ....

The hazards of working on this equipment/item have been explained to me and I agree to work within the guidelines

Signature... Name (printed)..

Company... Date ....

MANAGEMENT FORM

Figure 7.16 Form for declaration of contamination status and authorisation to work

DOCUMENTATION AND RECORDS

Previous sections have outlined a procedure for equipment management, an equipment inventory, and the use of a log book for specified purposes. However, the total documentation and records regarding the use of a particular instrument or piece of equipment involves other separate but interrelated sources. In the case of a microscope this might be quite simple and involve an entry in the equipment inventory with a record of maintenance contracts and the preparation of working instructions. In the case of an analyser such as the fictitious but nevertheless realistic **BHM** Analyser the situation is more complex. This analyser is based in the Biochemistry Department but is used by staff in **B**iochemistry, **H**aematology and **M**icrobiology to perform different analyses and Figure 7.17 illustrates all the documentation that may be involved in its management and operation.

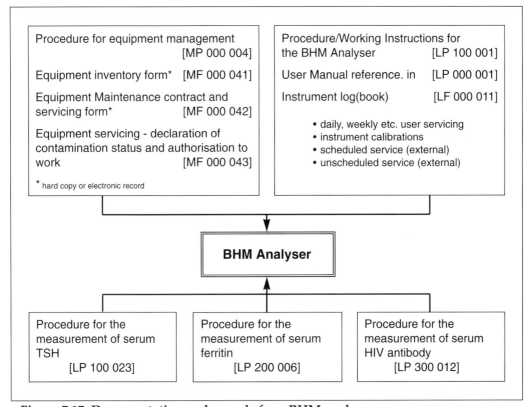

Figure 7.17 Documentation and records for a BHM analyser

Upon installation a record will be made on the equipment inventory form [MF 000 041]. After the period of warranty which is normally one year (with the exception of computer equipment which can be as little as ninety days), if appropriate an agreement for a servicing or maintenance contract is made and details entered on the servicing record [MF 000 042]. The details of such an agreement should be part of the initial purchasing discussions. The procedure/working instructions for the instrument [LP 000 001] should require that day to day details of 'in-house servicing' be kept in the instrument log [LF 000 011]. A record of instrument calibrations can also be kept in this log or alternatively on the appropriate work sheets which are created as a result of following the appropriate procedure, e.g. the procedure for the analysis of serum ferritin [LP 200 006]. Whether these records are kept in hard copy or electronic files does not matter, providing the records created are readily available for inspection and are stored in a secure manner.

1.0 General introduction	10.0 Maintenance (including decontamination)
2.0 Identification	11.0 Trouble shooting
3.0 Precautionary measures and warnings	12.0 Technical specification
4.0 Symbols	13.0 Supplementary information
	13.1 General
5.0 Installation	13.2 Brief operating instructions
5.1 General	13.3 List of uses and applications
5.2 Action upon delivery	13.4 Warranty limitations
5.3 Preparation prior to installation	13.5 Ordering information
5.4 Bringing into operation	13.6 Possibilities of extension
	13.7 Assistance
6.0 Theory	13.8 Supplementary theoretical information
7.0 Functions	
8.0 Performance criteria and limitations	
9.0 Operating procedure	
9.1 Preparation (including calibration)	
9.2 Measuring procedure	
9.3 Presentation of data	
9.4 Shut-down procedure	
9.5 Emergency analyses	
9.6 Internal quality control	
9.7 Special functions	
9.8 Disposal instructions	based upon EN 591:1994

Figure 7.18 Recommended content of a user manual

EQUIPMENT USER MANUALS

Figure 7.17 shows a user manual as part of the documentation for the BHM analyser and indicates that it is referred to in the Procedure/working instructions for the analyser. The user manual represents an important opportunity for manufacturers to establish themselves as quality providers. The provision of a quality user manual can save the laboratory a good deal of work in the preparation of necessary documentation. Some manufacturers also provide excellent logbooks which can be accepted as part of a laboratories documentation provided that its use is referred to in the operating procedure for the analyser. In 1994 CEN published a standard EN 591:1994 'In vitro diagnostic systems - Requirements for in vitro diagnostic instruments for professional use'. This standard includes a recommended content of a user manual, the headlines of which are given in Figure 7.18. The content of a user manual shown in Figure 7.18 shows a bias towards measuring equipment but it could very easily be adapted to other equipment, such as staining machines or microtomes in histopathology or to a plate pouring machine in microbiology. It provides a good framework against which to judge users manuals to ensure that they contain all the information required.

PROCEDURE FOR EQUIPMENT MANAGEMENT AND CALIBRATION

The content of a procedure for equipment management [MP 000 004] is shown in Figure 7.19. It covers a range of activities, some of which would be dealt with by the laboratory and some such as ordering equipment done in accordance with the standing orders of the parent body or host organisation. Reference to other figures in this chapter are given for further information.

Content of procedure	References to figures in this chapter
1.0 Purpose and Scope	*(Figure 7.13)*
2.0 Responsibility	
3.0 References	
4.0 Definitions	
5.0 Documentation	
6.0 Action and methods	
6.1 Assessment and justification of need	
6.2 Selection of equipment	
6.3 Acceptance procedure	
6.4 Training	
6.5 Documentation (including user manual)	*(Figure 7.18)*
6.5 Servicing (maintenance, repair and modification) including decontamination prior to servicing and permit to work	*(Figure 7.16)*
6.6 Disposal and replacement	
6.7 Establishment and maintenance of an equipment inventory	*(Figure 7.14 & 7.15)*

Figure 7.19 Content of procedure for equipment management

REQUIREMENTS FOR EQUIPMENT MANAGEMENT AND CALIBRATION

The requirements for equipment management and calibration in the different quality and accreditation schemes are shown in Figure 7.20.

System	Equipment (management and calibration)
ISO 9001:1994	**4. Quality system requirements** **4.9 Process control** 'The supplier shall identify and plan the production, installation and servicing processes which directly affect quality and shall ensure that these processes are carried out under controlled conditions.' b) Use of suitable production, installation and servicing equipment .... e) The approval of processes and equipment, as appropriate; g) Suitable maintenance of equipment to ensure continuing process capability **4.11 Control of inspection, measuring and test equipment** **4.11.1 *General*** 'The supplier shall establish and maintain documented procedures to control, calibrate and maintain inspection, measuring and test equipment (including test software) used by the supplier to demonstrate the conformance of product to the specified requirements. Inspection, measuring and test equipment shall be used in a manner which ensures that the measurement uncertainty is known and is consistent with the required measurement capability...'
EN 45001:1989	**5. Technical competence** **5.3 Premises and Equipment** **5.3.1 *Availability*** 'The testing laboratory shall be furnished with all items of equipment required for correct performance of the tests and measurements ....' **5.3.3 *Equipment*** 'All equipment shall be properly maintained. Details of maintenance procedures shall be available.........' '.............Measuring and testing equipment used in the testing laboratory shall be calibrated where appropriate before being put into service and thereafter according to an established programme. ....'
OECD - GLP	**4. Apparatus, material and reagents** **4.1 Apparatus** (1) Apparatus used for the generation of data, and for controlling environmental factors relevant to the study should be suitably located and of appropriate design and adequate capacity. (2) Apparatus used in a study should be periodically inspected, cleaned, maintained, and calibrated according to Standard Operating Procedures. Records of procedures should be maintained.
CAP - LAP	**Standard II Resources and facilities** 'The pathology services shall have sufficient and appropriate space, equipment . . . for the performance of the volume of work .....' under the interpretative notes it says 'The scope of the responsibilities and activities of the pathology service must be delineated. Once this determination has been made, sufficient and appropriate space and equipment must be provided'.

CPA(UK)Ltd	**C Facilities and Equipment**
	C7 The laboratory equipment meets the demands of the service and is properly maintained
	D Policies and Procedures
	D11 There are written procedures for the regular maintenance of equipment

Figure 7.20   Requirements for equipment management and calibration

FURTHER READING

BS 7750:1994 Specification for Environmental management systems, British Standards Institute.

EN 591:1994 User manuals for in vitro diagnostic instruments for professional use, CEN.

Foster N. EC Law, 2nd Edition 1995, Blackstone Press Ltd, London.

Foster N. Blackstone's EC Legislation, 6th Edition 1995, Blackstone Press Ltd, London.

Hunter W Safety and health at work - Community initiatives since the Single European Act, 1987 Social Europe 3/93 Europe for safety and health at work; Health and Safety Directorate of the Directorate-General for Employment, Industrial Relations and Social Affairs of the European Commission.

Inspection checklist, Anatomic Pathology and Cytology, 1995.1, Section VIII, College of American Pathologists.

Laboratory Assessment Checklist, 1981. Anatomical Pathology, Commonwealth Department of Health National Pathology Accreditation Advisory Council.

Laboratory Assessment Checklist, 1981. Blood banking, blood grouping and cross matching; Commonwealth Department of Health National Pathology Accreditation Advisory Council.

Management of Medical equipment and devices, January 1991; Health Equipment Information, Department of Health (UK).

Safe working and the prevention of infection in the mortuary and post-mortem room, 1991. Health Services Advisory Committee, Health and Safety Commission, HSE Books, Sudbury, UK.

The Patient's Charter, National Health Service, 1991, Department of Health (UK).

Workplace health, safety and welfare, 1992; Approved code of practice and guidance on regulations, Health and Safety Executive.

Chapter 8

Health and safety

INTRODUCTION

The introduction to the previous chapter should serve in part as an introduction to the present chapter. It established by reference to the EC 'framework directive' the principles with regard to health and safety in the workplace (Figure 7.3). Whilst Chapter 7 looked at aspects of facilities in terms of premises and equipment this chapter focuses on the organisation and management of health and safety. It is not intended to be an authoritative guide to all aspects of the subject. The Further Reading provided will give valuable information particularly when read in conjunction with the legislation of a particular country.

ORGANISATION AND MANAGEMENT

HEALTH AND SAFETY POLICY

In many countries it is a legal requirement that every employer (except where less than five people are employed) must prepare and, as often as may be appropriate, revise a written statement of the general policy with respect to the health and safety at work of employees, of any other person entering the workplace, and of the organisation and arrangements for carrying out that policy. This statement and any revisions must be brought to the attention of all employees. The policy statement of St Elsewhere's Hospital Trust is shown in Figure 8.1. This general policy statement forms the first item in the Health and Safety Handbook, and would be referred to in the purpose and scope of the laboratory procedure for the organisation and management of health and safety. In the arrangements described in this chapter this procedure requires the preparation of a Health and Safety Handbook which is a major vehicle for communication to employees.

RESPONSIBILITIES

EMPLOYER/MANAGEMENT

The EC 'framework directive' has a general provision that the employer has the overall responsibility for health and safety in the workplace and Article 6 which deals with general obligations for employers says '...the employer shall take measures necessary for the

---

The Health and Safety Policy of St Elsewhere's Hospital Trust

1. The Trust recognises that the safety of all its employees and other persons on its premises is of paramount importance and accepts its responsibility for providing a safe and healthy workplace.

2. The Trust will meet its responsibility, so far as is reasonably practical, paying particular attention to the provision and maintenance of:
   - a safe place of work with safe access to and from it.
   - a healthy working environment.
   - plant, equipment and systems of work which are safe.
   - safe arrangements for the use, handling, storage and transport of articles and substances.
   - sufficient information, instruction, training and supervision to enable employees to avoid hazards and contribute positively to their own health and safety at work.

3. The Trust undertakes the systematic identification of hazards, the recording of any significant risks arising from them, the establishment of arrangements to eliminate, reduce or control risks, and procedures for the review and revision of these arrangements.

4. The Trust will appoint safety officers competent to provide health and safety advice and assistance and to deal with emergencies and situations of imminent danger to health and safety.

5. The Trust will co-operate fully in the appointment of safety representatives and will provide them, where necessary, with sufficient facilities and training to carry out this task.

6. The Trust will ensure the existence of a Health and Safety Committee.

7. A copy of this statement will be brought to the attention of all employees. It will be reviewed, or modified from time to time and may be supplemented in appropriate cases by further statements relating to the work of particular groups of employees.

Signature of The Chief Executive and date

The Chief Executive of St Elsewhere's Hospital Trust

Figure 8.1 The health and safety policy of St Elsewhere's Hospital Trust

safety and health protection of workers, including the prevention of occupational risks and provision of information and training, as well as provision of the necessary organisation and means'.

Although the overall organisation and management of health and safety lies with the employer, the successful implementation and maintenance of any policy depends on co-operation of all the personnel in the laboratory. An understanding of the responsibilities of the different parties is extremely important, and includes, in addition to the employer, the employees' representative(s), the workers or employees, and the Health and Safety Officer. Each member of staff should have a clear reporting line with regard to health and safety matters. The parent body or host organisation may also have a Fire Officer or advice from the local fire service, trained first aiders and an occupational health department.

WORKERS REPRESENTATIVE

Article 11 of the EC 'framework directive' on consultation (with) and participation (of) workers states that 'employers shall consult workers and/or their representatives and allow them to take part in discussions on all questions relating to safety and health at work' and requires employers among other things, to allow 'adequate time off work, without loss of pay, and provide them with the necessary means to enable such representatives to exercise their rights and functions deriving from the Directive'. Such representatives have a valuable role to play in any well run laboratory. They could be members of the Health and Safety Committee or report to it.

WORKERS/EMPLOYEES

In most legislation on health and safety not only does the employer/management have the overall responsibility but also the workers themselves have responsibilities. Article 13 of the 'framework directive' says 'It shall be the responsibility of each worker to take care as far as possible of his* own safety and health and that of other persons affected by his acts or omissions at work in accordance with his training and instructions given by his employer'. To this end it requires workers to make correct use of work equipment and personal protective equipment, to have due regard to safety devices, to co-operate with the employer or worker representatives and to inform them of any work situation that they consider to represent a serious and immediate danger to health and safety.

LABORATORY SAFETY OFFICER

In Article 7, Protective and preventative services, it states that the 'employer shall designate one or more workers to carry out activities related to the protection and prevention of occupational risks for the undertaking and/or establishment'. Alternatively in the absence of competent personnel 'the employer shall enlist competent external services or persons'. Pathology laboratories should have a designated safety officer or officers. It is important that all staff understand the role of the safety officer and where it begins and ends (Figure 8.2). In particular it is important to understand that diminution or termination of risk is a management responsibility.

---

*The wording of the directive uses 'his' but it would read better as 'their' and 'the' as appropriate.

A laboratory safety officer should be appointed by management...

- to provide guidance to management and supervisors.
- to propose a safety programme and provide safety expertise.
- to propose, provide or obtain safety and training.
- to serve ex *officio* on the health and safety committee.
- to carry out risk assessments and recommend action as required.
- to stop activities that are unsafe and be authorised by management to do so.

...but diminution or termination of risk is a management responsibility

---

Figure 8.2   The laboratory safety officer

HEALTH AND SAFETY COMMITTEE

An important way in which to co-ordinate all health and safety matters is by having a Health and Safety Committee. The chairman could either be the Director of Pathology or a senior person to whom the responsibility is delegated. Its primary function will be to ensure that procedures for the organisation and management of health and safety are implemented. The Laboratory Safety Officer is an important member of the Health and Safety Committee but may be able to function better by having an advisory/reporting role rather than being chairman of the committee. In addition to workers representatives, the committee should have representatives from each department in pathology so that all issues are represented. Although the committee has the important role of co-ordination, every individual member of staff must understand their responsibilities which must form part of their job descriptions (see Figures 6.5 and 6.6).

DOCUMENTATION

THE LABORATORY HEALTH AND SAFETY HANDBOOK

The term 'handbook' is used deliberately in this section to distinguish it from the manuals which form part of the overall structure of the Quality Manual (see Figure 4.2). Nevertheless the responsibility for its production and updating should be clearly defined in section 6.3.1 of the Organisation and Management procedure (Figure 8.11) and be subject to the document control procedures described in Chapter 4.

The Trust Health and Safety Policy

1 Maintenance and Inspection of the Laboratory for Safety

   1.1   Organisation and responsibilities
   1.2   Procedures
   1.3   Records
   1.4   Risk assessment
   1.5   Incident reporting

2 General requirements for Personal and Laboratory Safety

   2.1   Smoking
   2.2   Food and drink
   2.3   Cosmetics
   2.4   Hair, beards and jewellery
   2.5   Hand washing

   2.6   Eye and face protection
   2.7   Eye wash
   2.8   Protective clothing
   2.9   Shoes
   2.10 Emergency showers
   2.11 Respirators

   2.12 Mouth pipetting
   2.13 Sharp objects
   2.14 Isolation procedures
   2.15 Glassware
   2.16 Centrifuges
   2.17 Good housekeeping

3 First aid provision

4 Bomb threats

5 Fire prevention and control

6 Warning signs and labels

7 Electrical safety

8 Compressed gases

9 Chemical hazards

10 Carcinogens

11 Microbiological hazards

12 Radiation safety

13 Reports of accidents, illness and incidents

14 Waste management

Appendix - Floor plan of laboratory showing:-

- Fire exits
- Fire extinguishers and hose reels
- Alarm indicator board
- Emergency shower
- First aid boxes
- Contact numbers
- Eyewash stations
- Handwash basins
- Toilets

Figure 8.3   Content of a laboratory health and safety handbook

Figure 8.3 provides a framework for creating a Health and Safety Handbook for the laboratory (often called the Laboratory Safety Handbook). The detailed content will be partly determined by local rules, guidelines, codes of practice, and regulations. In many countries the governmental organisations responsible for the inspection of health, safety and welfare in the workplace produce valuable informative literature regarding the handling of certain situations. The style of presentation and accessibility of the handbook is important if it is to be used for the education and training of staff and management. The Health and Safety Policy statement could either be that of the laboratory or of the parent body or host organisation. All new employees are required to read the handbook as part of their induction training and informally examined as to their understanding (see Figure 6.9).

In the UK the Health Service Advisory Committee of the UK Health and Safety Commission has produced a series of model rules for staff and visitors which could be included in the Health and Safety handbook as appendices or as free standing posters. They include model rules for clinical, scientific, technical and medical laboratory staff, phlebotomists and venepuncturists, laboratory office staff, laboratory reception staff, laboratory porters and messengers, cleaning staff in the laboratory (domestic and ancillary), maintenance staff and equipment service engineers in clinical laboratories, and for visitors to laboratories. As an example the model rules for laboratory office staff are shown in Figure 8.4.

Rules for laboratory office staff

Most of the work in the laboratory is concerned with the handling of specimens that may be infectious. Office staff are not required to come into direct contact with these materials but may accidentally do so when handling bags and packages containing specimens. Such workers, in addition to following the general precautions outlined above, should also take the following safety measures.

(a) If you work in an office that has direct access into the laboratory, wear a coat or gown, like the other laboratory staff.

(b) Wash your hands after you have been into the laboratory and may have come into contact with laboratory items or materials that could be infectious.

(c) Never lick stamps or labels. User a roller pad, damp sponge or self-adhesive labels.

(d) If you are required to package specimens, only do so if the containers are in a sealed transport bag. If there is any sign of breakage or leakage do not touch the bag. Report it to your supervisor immediately.

'Safe working and the prevention of infection in clinical laboratories - model rules for staff and visitors'
Health Service Advisory Committee of the Health and Safety Commission (UK) 1991.

Figure 8.4   Model rules for laboratory office staff

The NCCLS Document M29-T2 'Protection of Laboratory Workers from Infectious Disease Transmitted by Blood, Body Fluids and Tissue' contains a valuable summary of recommendations (see Figure 8.5).

Protection of Laboratory Workers from Infectious Diseases Transmitted by Blood, Body Fluids, and Tissue

Summary of Recommendations (NCCLS Document M29-T2)

Universal precautions

1. Barrier protection at all times.
2. Gloves for blood and body fluids. Gloves in volunteer donor sites optional.
3. Phlebotomist wears gloves:
   - With uncooperative patient.
   - With non-intact skin.
   - When performing skin puncture.
   - When in training.
4. Change gloves between patients.
5. Facial protection from splashing.
6. Gown and apron for splashes.
7. Wash hands if contaminated.
8. Wash hands after removing gloves.
9. Avoid accidental injuries.
10. Rigid needle containers.
11. Don't handle needles.
12. Reprocess sharps carefully.
13. No mouth-to-mouth resuscitation contact.
14. Minimise spills and spatters.
15. Decontaminate all surfaces and devices after use.

Protection Techniques

1. Wash hands after contamination, removing gloves, and work.
2. Wear gloves; change after contamination.
3. Full face shield, or goggles and mask for spatter.
4. Occlusive bandages as needed.
5. Wear gown/lab coat always; apron as needed.
6. Use personal respirator if risk of aerosolised M.tuberculosis is present.

Decontamination of spills

1. Tuberculocidal hospital disinfectant.
   - Wear gloves and gown.
   - Absorb spill.
   - Clean with detergent.
   - 1:10 dilution bleach.
   - Wash with water.
   - Biohazard disposal

Laboratory Procedures

1. Biosafety level 2.
2. No warning labels.
3. Reduce needles/syringes.
4. No mouth pipetting.
5. Leakproof primary and secondary containers.
6. Use centrifuge safety cups.
7. Use biohazard disposal techniques.
   - Infectious waste in "Red Bag".
   - "Red Bag" in rigid container.
   - Sharps in rigid container.
   - Proper storage, transport, and disposal of waste.
8. Service personnel follow universal precautions.
9. "One handed" technique with evacuated tube adapters.

Accidents

HBV - HB vaccine + HGIB if high risk source.

HIV - In clinical setting:

   Voluntary HIV antibody test from source and worker.

   - In laboratory setting:

   Test source specimen and worker.

Consider AZT prophylaxis within one hour of exposure. 200 mg every 6 hours. Follow-up 1, 2, 3 and 6 months.

The Autopsy

1. May modify universal precautions.
2. Circulator recommended.
3. Barrier protection:
   - Head-to-toe fluid resistant garb and apron.
   - Double gloves/Heavy-duty gloves/Stainless steel mesh gloves.
4. Procedures:
   - Modified Rokitansky or Virchow evisceration.
   - Confine all contaminated materials to autopsy table or photo-stand.
   - One scalpel blade at table.
   - One prosector.
   - Fix all tissues at table.
   - No frozen sections.
   - Decontaminate completely.

Surgical Specimens

1. Follow universal precautions.
2. Use gloves for frozen sections.

Regulatory Compliance

- Administrative - Develop SOPs.
- Training and education.
- Engineering controls.
- Safe work practices.
- Personal protective equipment.
- Medical - HB vaccine.
- Record keeping.

See NCCLS Guideline I17-P, Protection of Laboratory Workers from Instrument Biohazards.

Figure 8.5   Summary of recommendations (NCCLS Document M29-T2)

Permission to reproduce this Summary from M29-T2 (Protection of laboratory workers from infectious disease transmitted by blood, body fluids, and tissue - Second Edition; Tentative Guideline) has been granted by NCCLS. This Summary highlights recommendations described in detail in M29-T2. Users of this summary should have M29-T2 available, and should be familiar with the recommendations it contains (see Appendix 1 for address).

FORMS AND CHECKLISTS

The forms and checklists used in risk assessment, monitoring, audit and incident reporting are described in the appropriate sections below. It is these completed forms and checklists, together with the minutes of the Health and Safety Committee, that represent the records which can be referred to at a quality or accreditation inspection to establish compliance with the stated policy.

RISK ASSESSMENT

The process of risk assessment requires the identification of hazards. They can arise from the activities taking place in the laboratory or from other factors such as the layout of the laboratory. A *hazard* can be defined as 'something with the potential to do harm, and include for example, chemical substances, biological agents, equipment or methods of working'. The term *risk* is 'the likelihood that some harm can come from the particular hazard', and the *'extent of risk'* means the number of people who might be exposed to the hazard and the consequences for them.

Article 6 of the ECC 'framework directive' includes among the general obligations on employers the requirement that they shall 'evaluate the risks to the safety and health of the workers, *inter alia* in the choice of work equipment, the chemical substances or preparation used, and the fitting out of work places'. The requirement to evaluate risks to workers is a continuing theme in subsequent directives issued under the 'framework directive' and includes directives on 'Use of work equipment' (Directive 89/655/EEC of 30 November 1989), 'Use of personal protective equipment' (Directive 89/656/EEC of 30 November 1989), Use of display screen equipment' (Directive 90/270/EEC of 29 May 1990 and the 'Manual handling of loads' (Directive 90/269/EEC of 29 May 1990), all of which have application in the pathology laboratory. In most countries there are also regulations concerning the use of chemical and biological agents, carcinogens (including a prohibition list) and radioisotopes (*in vitro* and *in vivo*). In all these areas not only is an evaluation of the risks to workers required but also workers must receive the results of the risk assessments. The hazards to be evaluated can range from a filing cabinet being unstable with the drawers open, to the handling of samples which might contain HIV.

In the EC and in other legislatures the evaluation of risk is a legal requirement. If an employer has difficulty in understanding how to undertake risk evaluations, the local Health and Safety Inspectorate can provide information on relevant publications. The Health and Safety Executive (UK) has prepared a leaflet to guide the process entitled 'Five steps to risk assessment'. It is important for whoever is undertaking the risk assessment, whether it is the employer or a person designated to do it on their behalf such as a Health and Safety Officer or an outside expert, to follow the steps recommended.

As this concept of risk assessment is becoming increasingly important, particularly with regard to acceptance for insurance, further advice regarding each step is summarised in Figure 8.6.

Step 1 Look for the hazards

♦ Walk around your laboratory and look afresh at what could reasonably be expected to cause harm.
♦ Ignore the trivial and concentrate on significant hazards which could result in serious harm or affect several people.
♦ Ask your employees or their representatives what they think. They may have noticed things which are not immediately obvious.
♦ Manufacturer's instructions or datasheets can also help you spot hazards and put risks in their true perspective. So can accident and ill-health records.

Step 2 Decide who might be harmed, and how

♦ As well as people who work in the laboratory all the time, think about people who work there occasionally, e.g. cleaners, visitors, contractors, maintenance personnel, etc.
♦ Include members of the public if there is a chance they could be hurt by your activities.

Step 3 Evaluate the risks arising from the hazards and decide whether existing precautions are adequate or more should be done

♦ Even after all precautions have been taken, usually some risk remains. What you have to decide for each significant hazard is whether this remaining risk is high, medium or low.
♦ First, ask yourself whether you have done all the things that the law or a code of good practice says you have got to do, e.g. guidance regarding the wearing of protective clothing whilst using disinfectants in mortuaries.
♦ Then ask yourself whether generally accepted standards are in place, e.g. provision of protective clothing and training in its use.
♦ But don't stop there - think about yourself as an employer, because the law also says that you must do what is reasonably practicable to keep your laboratory safe.
♦ Your real aim is to make all risks small by adding to your precautions if necessary.

Step 4 Record your findings

♦ You must record the significant findings of your assessment by (1) writing down the more significant hazards and (2) recording your most important conclusions,
e.g. Use of disinfectants in mortuary: protective clothing provided and training given.
♦ You must also inform your employees about your findings.
♦ Assessments need to be suitable and sufficient, not perfect. The real points are: are the precautions reasonable, and is there something to show that a proper check was made?
♦ Keep the written document for future reference or use; it can help you if an inspector questions your precautions, or if you become involved in any action for civil liability. It can also remind you to keep an eye on particular matters. And it helps to show that you have done what the law requires.
♦ To make things simpler, you can refer to other documents, such as manuals, the arrangements in your health and safety policy statement, manufacturer's instructions, and your health and safety procedures.

Step 5 Review your assessment from time to time and revise it if necessary

♦ Sooner or later you will bring in new apparatus, substances and procedures which could lead to new hazards. You should add to the assessment to take account of the new hazard.
♦ It is good practice to review your assessment from time to time.
♦ Don't amend your assessment for every trivial change, or still more, for each new activity, but if a new activity introduces significant new hazards of its own, you will want to consider them in their own right and do whatever you need to keep the risks down.

adapted from '5 steps to Risk Assessment'. Health and Safety Executive (1994)

Figure 8.6 Five steps to risk assessment

ACCIDENT AND INCIDENT REPORTING

Even when effective risk assessment has been completed in a laboratory and the appropriate steps have been taken to minimise the risk associated with the hazards identified, inevitably there will still be incidents such as 'needle stick' injuries. It is an important part of health and safety procedure that these incidents are recorded and an investigation carried out to determine whether the risk can be further reduced. This may require changes in particular procedures or improvements in the training given to staff.

One of the major problems with all aspects of health and safety is how to maintain interest in a topic which staff may regard as an extra imposition on an already busy day. How often do laboratory staff attend fire lectures with enthusiasm!

All incidents should be recorded and evaluated as part of the health and safety procedure but additionally in many countries there is a legal requirement to report certain injuries, diseases and dangerous occurrences to the appropriate enforcing authority for record and, if appropriate, investigation. Which incidents constitute reportable events will differ in different countries but Figure 8.7 shows a typical categorisation with examples which are appropriate to a laboratory situation.

MONITORING AND AUDIT

The process of risk assessment has similarities with monitoring and audit. However, monitoring and audit have more to do with compliance with the advised precautionary measures, for example laboratory staff wearing protective clothing when appropriate, as distinct from the provision of protective clothing as a response to a risk assessment. A comprehensive safety audit should be conducted at least annually and the report presented to workers/representatives and the Pathology Management Board. The minutes of the Board should record acceptance of the audit and the response to any recommendations. In order that nothing of importance is missed audits are best carried out against a check list which can also serve to provide a record of the audit. A useful basis for a check list can be the contents of the Laboratory Safety Handbook or the laboratory safety sections of inspection checklists of accreditation schemes (e.g. CAP-LAP) or the requirements with which employers have to comply in relation to particular legislation. In the CAP-LAP Inspection Checklist - Laboratory General, Section I, questions are included on the general safety programme for the whole laboratory. It is divided into two sections; the first involves questions concerning 'manuals and records', and the second the 'physical inspection of the laboratory'. A selection of questions from both sections is shown in Figure 8.8, and Figure 8.9 shows the first page of a Health and Safety Audit form used in pathology at St Elsewhere's Hospital Trust which is based on this material.

Death or major injury

An accident connected with work and where your employee, or a self-employed person working on your premises, is killed or suffers a major injury (including as a result of physical violence); or a member of the public is killed or taken to hospital, e.g.

- unconsciousness caused by asphyxia or exposure to harmful substance or biological agent;
- acute illness requiring medical treatment, or loss of consciousness arising from absorption of any substance by inhalation, ingestion or through the skin;
- Acute illness requiring medical treatment where there is reason to believe that this resulted from exposure to a biological agent or its toxins or infected material.

Over-three day injury

An accident connected with work (including an act of physical violence) and your employee, or a self-employed person working on your premises, suffers an over-three-day injury. An over-three-day injury is one which is not major but results in the injured person being away from work or unable to do their normal work for more than three days (including non work days).

Disease

If a doctor notifies you that your employee suffers from a reportable work-related disease. Definitions e.g.

- certain poisonings;
- some skin diseases such as occupational dermatitis, skin cancer, chrome ulcer, oil folliculitis/acne;
- infections such as: leptospirosis; hepatitis; tuberculosis; anthrax; legionellosis and tetanus

Dangerous occurrence

If something happens which does not result in a reportable injury, but which clearly could have done, then it may be a dangerous occurrence which must be reported, e.g.

- accidental release of a biological agent likely to cause severe human illness;
- accidental release of any substance which may damage health.

adapted from Reporting of injuries, Diseases and Dangerous Occurrences regulations
Health and Safety Executive (1996)

Figure 8.7   Categories of reportable incidents

Monitoring should be seen as an ongoing formal or informal process of checking compliance to understood and promulgated standards. It might for example involve gentle but firm reminders to heads of departments that they too should wear protective clothing in the 'dirty' areas of the laboratory! In addition to internal monitoring and audit, inspectors from the appropriate Government Agency will make visits from time to time and present a report in which any non compliances to regulations or codes of practice are listed. The employer/management will have to respond in a given period and satisfy the inspectorate that remedial action has been taken. Occasionally a non compliance might be serious enough to require immediate suspension of a particular activity.

Manuals and records

1. Are safety policies and procedures posted or readily available to all personnel?
2. Have policies and procedures been developed regarding the documentation of all laboratory accidents resulting in property damage or involving spillage of hazardous substances?
3. Have policies and procedures been developed regarding the reporting of all occupational injuries or illnesses that require medical treatment (more than first aid)?
4. Have an evaluation of these incident and accident reports been incorporated into the laboratory's quality improvement program to avoid recurrence?
5. Are policies and procedures documented and adequate for fire prevention and control?
6. Are fire drills conducted quarterly?
7. Have personnel been instructed in the use of portable fire extinguishers?
8. Are policies and procedures documented and adequate for the safe handling of electrical equipment? Are policies and procedures documented and adequate for chemical toxin hazard control?
9. Is there documentation that each of the chemicals in the laboratory has been evaluated for carcinogenic potential, reproductive toxicity, and acute toxicity; and does the policies and procedure manual define specific handling requirements for these chemicals?
10. Are policies and procedures documented and adequate for hazardous waste disposal?

Physical inspection of the laboratory

1. Is the laboratory properly separated from in-patient areas and/or provided with automatic fire extinguishing (AFE) systems?
2. Is there an automatic fire detection and alarm system?
3. Is the fire alarm audible in all parts of the laboratory, including storage areas, lavatories, and darkrooms?
4. Are appropriate fire extinguishers provided for all areas in which flammable and combustible liquids are stored or handled?
5. Is emergency lighting adequate for safe evacuation of the laboratory?
6. Is there documentation that all laboratory instruments and appliances are adequately grounded and checked for current leakage at least every 12 months?
7. Are supplies of flammable and combustible liquids reasonable for the laboratory's needs, and are they properly stored?
8. Are storage areas and/or rooms where volatile solvents are used adequately ventilated?
9. Are flammable or combustible liquids or gas cylinders positioned well away from open flame or other heat sources, not in corridors and not within exhaust canopies?
10. Are flammable-gas cylinders stored in a separate, ventilated room or enclosure, reserved exclusively for that purpose, and which has a fire-resistance classification of at least two hours?

Source CAP-LAP Inspection Checklist, Laboratory General I 1995.1

Figure 8.8   Items for health and safety audit

EDUCATION AND TRAINING

An important part of creating a good 'health and safety culture' is the education and training provided. Any courses attended by members of staff should be recorded in their personnel record (see Figure 6.7). The important factor in education and training is to make it relevant to the individual's particular situation. If a member of staff has to move heavy gas cylinders then for that individual a course in manual handling would be relevant and meaningful. A useful approach is to design material that encourages members of staff to evaluate their own work situation and Government Agencies responsible for

St Elsewhere's Hospital Trust

PATHOLOGY

MF 000 051
Edition 1
Page 1/5

HEALTH AND SAFETY AUDIT FORM

Location

Department ....

Room or locality ....

Section 1.0   Manuals and methods

1.1 Are safety policies and procedures posted or readily available to all personnel?   **(YES   NO   N/A)**

If answer is no, please record comment below

1.2 Have policies and procedures been developed regarding the documentation of all laboratory accidents resulting in property damage or involving spillage of hazardous substances?   **(YES   NO   N/A)**

If answer is no, please record comment below

1.3 Have policies and procedures been developed regarding the reporting of all occupational injuries or illnesses that require medical treatment (more than first aid) ?   **(YES   NO   N/A)**

If answer is no, please record comment below

1.4 Has an evaluation of these incident and accident reports been incorporated into the laboratory's quality improvement programme to avoid recurrence?   **(YES   NO   N/A)**

If answer is no, please record comment below

MANAGEMENT FORM

Figure 8.9   Model health and safety audit form

Health and Safety often have useful material available. A good example is a pamphlet, 'Working with VDUs', produced by the Health and Safety Executive (UK) which provides information concerning the UK regulations which were developed in response to ECC Directive 90/270/EEC of 29 May 1990, on 'Use of display screen equipment'. In addition to answering questions about health matters it outlines the regulations and what employers have to do to comply, and finishes with a section entitled 'What can I do to help myself?'(Figure 8.10).

WHAT CAN I DO TO HELP MYSELF?

Lots! You should make full use of the adjustment facilities for your VDU and work environment to get the best from them and avoid potential health problems. If the Regulations apply to you, your employer must cover these things in training. If the Regulations don't apply to you, using these facilities is still important. Here are some specific tips.

1. Adjust your chair and VDU to find the most comfortable position for your work. As a broad guide, your arms should be approximately horizontal and your eyes at the same height as the top of the VDU casing.

2. Make sure there is enough space underneath your desk to move your legs freely. Move any obstacles such as boxes or equipment.

3. Avoid excess pressure on the backs of your legs and knees. A footrest, particularly for smaller users, may be helpful.

4. Don't sit in the same position for long periods. Make sure you change your posture as often as practicable. Some movement is desirable, but avoid repeat stretching movements.

5. Adjust your keyboard and screen to get a good keying and viewing position. A space in front of the keyboard is sometimes helpful for resting the hands and wrists while not keying.

6. Don't bend your hands up at the wrist when keying. Try to keep a soft touch on the keys and don't overstretch your fingers. Good keyboard technique is important.

7. Try different layouts of keyboard, screen and document holder to find the best arrangement for you.

8. Make sure you have enough work space to take whatever documents you need. A document holder may help you to avoid awkward neck movements.

9. Arrange your desk and screen so that bright lights are not reflected on the screen. You shouldn't be directly facing windows or bright lights. Adjust curtains or blinds to prevent unwanted light.

10. Make sure the characters on your screen are sharply focused and can be read easily. They shouldn't flicker or move.

11. Make sure there are no layers of dirt, grime or finger marks on the screen. Use the brightness control on the screen to suit the lighting conditions in the room.

from Working with VDUs, Health and Safety Executive (1995)

Figure 8.10 Use of display screen equipment - What can I do to help myself?'

PROCEDURE FOR THE ORGANISATION AND MANAGEMENT OF HEALTH AND SAFETY

The content of a procedure for the organisation and management of health and safety in the pathology laboratory of St Elsewhere's' Hospital Trust is shown in Figure 8.11. Certain issues will be developed in concert with the parent body or host organisation but the majority of the issues will be peculiar to the laboratory.

Content of the procedure	References to other figures in the text
1.0 Purpose and scope	*(Figure 8.1 Health and safety policy of parent body)*
2.0 Responsibilities	
3.0 References	
4.0 Definitions	
5.0 Documents	
6.0 Actions and Methods	
6.1 Organisation and management	*(Figure 7.3 for main principles)*
6.1.1 General 6.1.2 Management/employer 6.1.3 Workers representative(s) 6.1.4 Workers/employees 6.1.5 Health and Safety Officer	
6.2 Health and Safety Committee	*(Figure 8.2)*
6.2.1 Officers and membership 6.2.2 Frequency of meetings 6.2.3 Agenda 6.2.4 Minutes	
6.3 Documentation	
6.3.1 Health and Safety Handbook (including model rules) 6.3.2 Forms and records	*(Figures 8.3 and 8.4)*
6.4 Labelling of hazards	*(Figure 8.6)*
6.5 Risk assessment	*(Figure 8.7)*
6.6 Accident and incident reporting	*(Figure 8.8 and 8.9)*
6.7 Monitoring and Audit	*(Figure 8.10)*
6.8 Education and Training	

Figure 8.11 Contents of a procedure for the organisation and management of health and safety

REQUIREMENT FOR HEALTH, SAFETY AND WELFARE

The requirements for health, safety and welfare in the different quality and accreditation systems are shown in Figure 8.12.

System	Health, safety and welfare
ISO 9001:1994	**4. Quality system requirements** *(There are no explicit requirements for health and safety in this standard)*
EN 45001:1989	**5. Technical competence** **5.3 Premises and Equipment** *5.3.2 Premises and environment* '. . . . The testing premises shall be protected as required from excessive conditions such as heat, dust, moisture, steam, noise, vibration and electromagnetic disturbance or interference, and shall be maintained accordingly. They shall be sufficiently spacious to limit the risk of damage or danger and to allow operators to make practical and precise movements . . .' Access to and use of all test areas shall be controlled in a manner appropriate to their designated purpose and conditions of entry by persons external to the laboratory shall be defined. Adequate measures shall be taken to ensure good housekeeping in the testing laboratory.

OECD - GLP	**1. Test facility organisation and personnel**
	1.1 Management's Responsibilities
	(2) At a minimum it should :
	    (d) Ensure that health and safety precautions are applied according to national and/or international regulations;
	1.2 Personnel Responsibilities
	(1) Personnel should exercise safe working practice. Chemicals should be handled with suitable caution until their hazard(s) has been established.
	(2) Personnel should exercise health precautions to minimise risk to themselves and to ensure the integrity of the study.
	3. Facilities
	3.5 Waste disposal
	(2) The handling and disposal of wastes generated during the performance of a study should be carried out in a manner which is consistent with pertinent regulatory requirements. This would include provision for appropriate collection, storage, and disposal facilities, decontamination and transportation procedures, and the maintenance of records related to the preceding activities.
	7. Standard Operating Procedures
	7.2 Application
	(1) Standard Operating procedures should be available for, but not be limited to, the following categories of laboratory activities. The details given under each heading are to be considered as illustrative examples.
	    (f) Health and Safety Precautions
	    As required by national and/or international legislation or guidelines.

CAP - LAP	**Standard I Director and Personnel Requirements** under the interpretative notes it says **A Qualifications, responsibilities, and role of the Director** (15) **Safety responsibilities** - Promote a safe laboratory environment for personnel and other occupants **Standard II Resources and facilities** under the interpretative notes it says: 'The laboratory must be a safe working place for the personnel and for the patients it serves. It must comply with the safety codes of the regulatory authorities. The safe collection and handling of patient specimens and of reagents shall be an integral part of the laboratory safety program. Proper disposal of hazardous wastes must be provided.'
CPA(UK)Ltd	**C Facilities and Equipment** **C11** There is a safe working environment in accordance with current legislation. **D Policies and Procedures** **D11** There are written procedures for the regular maintenance of equipment under Guidelines it says 'where necessary permit workforms should be provided and signed'

Figure 8.12 Requirements for health and safety

FURTHER READING

CAP Inspection Checklist, Laboratory General: Section I in Health and Safety 1995.1, College of American Pathology Environmental Health and Safety Resource Committee.

Clinical Laboratory Safety; Approved Guideline 1996, NCCLS Document GP17-A.

Clinical Laboratory Waste Management; Approved Guideline 1993, NCCLS Document GP5-A.

Display screen equipment at work: Health and Safety (Display Screen Equipment) Regulations 1992, Guidance on Regulations, HSE Books, Sudbury, UK.

Everyone's guide to RIDDOR, 1995; Reporting of injuries, diseases and dangerous occurrences regulations, Health and Safety Executive.

Five steps to risk assessment, 1994; A step by step guide to a safer and healthier workplace, Health and Safety Executive.

Guidelines for preparation of manuals for administrative instructions and personnel procedures for laboratories, Commonwealth Department of Health, Australia, NPAAC

HIV and the Practice of Pathology, 1995; Report of the Working Party of the Royal College of Pathologists.

Manual handling: Manual Handling Operations Regulations 1992, Guidance on Regulations HSE Books, Sudbury, UK.

NCCLS Clinical Laboratory Safety 1996; Approved Guideline, NCCLS GP17-A.

Personal Protective equipment at work: Personal Protective Equipment at Work Regulations 1992, Guidance on Regulations, HSE Books, Sudbury, UK.

Protection of Laboratory Workers from Infectious Disease Transmitted by Blood, Body Fluids, and Tissue - Second Edition; Tentative Guideline 1991, NCCLS Document M29-T2.

Protection of Laboratory Workers from Instrument Biohazards; Proposed Guideline 1991, NCCLS Document I17-P.

Safe working and the prevention of infection in clinical laboratories - model rules for staff and visitors, 1991; Health Services Advisory Committee, HSE Books, Sudbury, UK.

Safe working and the prevention of infection in clinical laboratories, 1991; Health Services Advisory Committee, Safety in Health Service Laboratories, Health and Safety Commission.

Safe working and the prevention of infection in the mortuary and post-mortem room, 1991; Health Services Advisory Committee, Safety in Health Service Laboratories, Health and Safety Commission.

Work equipment: Provision and Use of Work Equipment Regulations 1992, Guidance on Regulations, HSE Books, Sudbury, UK.

Working with VDUs, April 1995; Health and Safety Executive.

Chapter 9

Operating process activities — preanalytical and postanalytical

INTRODUCTION

This chapter starts with a general introduction to the procedures and other documentation required for the operating process activities of the pathology laboratory. Such activities are sometimes thought of as starting when the specimen arrives in the laboratory with its request form and being completed when the report is dispatched from the laboratory. In this presentation a broader view will be taken with as much emphasis on the preanalytical and postanalytical phases of operating process activities as on the analytical phase. Some observers would describe the operating process activities as the 'total testing process' and have emphasised the importance of this 'holistic' approach by studies which indicate that of the mistakes occurring in laboratory testing in a 570-bed general and acute care hospital, 46% were attributed to the preanalytical, 7% to analytical and 47% to the postanalytical phases of testing, and that non-laboratory personnel accounted for 28.6% of these mistakes. As the CAP-LAP and CPA(UK)Ltd systems are designed for pathology laboratories, it is not difficult to identify which sections of the standards refer to the different phases of operating process activity. In other systems the parallel parts of the process are not so easy to determine and extra explanation is provided.

As well as the preanalytical and postanalytical phases, this chapter also covers the management and operation of laboratory computer systems. Laboratory computer systems have a major impact on all phases of operating activity processes, and procedures for the management and operation of laboratory computers are discussed. Chapter 10 focuses on the analytical phase and on the closely associated topic of the management and use of consumables, reagents, calibration and quality control material. Finally there is a section on near patient testing, representing as it does an operating process activity outside the laboratory and one in which the laboratory needs to participate in order that proper standards are maintained.

WHAT PROCEDURES ARE REQUIRED?

The term 'Brain-to-Brain Loop' was used by Lunberg some years ago to represent the interaction between clinicians and the laboratory, and identified a number of key stages in the process. In Figure 9.1 the stages in the 'Brain-to-Brain Loop' are identified with the preanalytical, analytical and postanalytical phases of operating process activities. In the right hand column the phases are divided into clearly defined steps, which can be regarded as the building blocks required when considering the need for operating process procedures. It will be seen that stage 7 of the 'Brain-to-Brain Loop' occurs in both the preanalytical and analytical phases. This is so that preparation in the sense of 'data acquisition from specimens and request forms' can be distinguished from preparation as 'specimen preparation'. Specimen preparation can range from the relatively simple procedure of separating serum from whole blood by centrifugation to complex processes in histopathology like 'cutting up' or 'gross examination' where it plays a major role in specimen analysis. In considering stages involving the pathology laboratory, it is important to

Phases in operating process activities	The stages in the 'Brain-to-Brain' loop	Steps in the operating process activities
PREANALYTICAL	1. Question 2. Test selection 3. Ordering ——————— 4. Identification 5. Collection 6. Transportation ——————— 7. Preparation	1. Doctor/patient consultation 2. Request form completed 3. Specimen collection 4. Specimen and request form transportation 5. Specimen and request form reception 6. Data acquisition from specimen and request form
ANALYTICAL	7. Preparation ——————— 8. Analysis	7. Specimen preparation 8. Specimen analysis
POSTANALYTICAL	9. Reporting 10. Interpretation ——————— 11. Physicians brain 12. Action	9. Reporting of results including interpretation and recommendations 10. Transmission of report 11. Receipt of report by the doctor, and consultation as appropriate

Figure 9.1   Different approaches to operating process activity

draw a distinction between clinical advice given by pathologists and senior scientific staff, and the situations in which pathologists have patients under their direct clinical care. In the latter case, stages 11 and 12 in the 'Brain-to-Brain Loop' would be involved but is outside the scope of this book. In all other stages the laboratory has a role. A valuable commentary on the 'Brain-to-Brain' loop will be found in Further Reading at the end of the chapter.

In deciding which procedures and other documentation will be required to adequately cover all operating process activities, it is necessary to consider the attributes which are associated with each step (see right hand column of Figure 9.1). These attributes can be posed as a series of questions: 'What does the step involve and why is it being done?', 'Where and when is it being done?', and finally 'Who does it and how?' Looking briefly at a general scenario in which a doctor requires a blood sample to be taken, an analysis to be performed and the result sent back to a specified location, the steps in the preanalytical phase must be examined to determine whether blood is to be taken in the doctor's office (general practitioner's surgery), in outpatients, on the wards, or in the phlebotomy suite of the pathology laboratory. The next consideration, which will partially be determined by where the blood is taken, is 'Who takes it?' It could be a doctor, nurse, phlebotomist or a member of the laboratory staff, and all may require training, particularly when a different system of collection is introduced. Finally, how does the specimen get to the laboratory, by courier, hospital porter, phlebotomist on the ward round, or by a pneumatic tube system, and how will it be received. Such an analysis may result in one or several written procedures being required depending on the way in which the laboratory is structured, one for specimen collection, one for training personnel to take blood, one for transportation, reception and data acquisition.

In Chapter 4 the structure of the documentation was described, and Figure 4.2 showed the structure of the quality manual with its four volumes of different procedure manuals. Any step in the preanalytical phase which involves participation of a patient requires a clinical procedure [CP 000 001 etc.] to be written (e.g. steps 1-3 in Figure 9.1). Any other step requires a laboratory procedure [LP 000 001]. Some of the procedures need to be discipline specific and some generic to pathology as a whole. Examples of clinical procedures such as dynamic function test procedures will be described in the clinical audit section of Chapter 11.

PREANALYTICAL

QUESTION, TEST SELECTION AND ORDERING

The importance of the provision of consultant advice as part of a laboratory service is made clear in the description of a laboratory service given in Figure 5.3. The way in which a doctor formulates the need for a test and then chooses the correct test will depend firstly on the reason for the request, secondly on their training in the use of the laboratory, and thirdly on the information provided by the laboratory.

There are a number of reasons why laboratory tests are ordered (Figure 9.2) and all medical staff on arrival in the hospital should, as part of their induction programme, be provided with information on the use of the laboratory and encouraged to visit the laboratory to meet the senior staff. As junior medical staff have an enormous amount of information to digest in their first few days at a new hospital, the information needs to be presented in a clear and easily accessible format.

- Diagnosis of disease
- Screening for disease
- Determination of disease severity
- Determination of patient management

- Monitoring of disease progress
- Detection and monitoring of drug toxicity
- Prediction of response to treatment

Figure 9.2   Reasons for ordering laboratory tests

In the NPAAC's Guidelines for the preparation of Laboratory Manuals it says 'the achievement of a consultative service ...can be aided by the preparation of a laboratory handbook for use by clinicians and staff requiring authoritative advice'. The title of the handbook is important and the term 'users handbook' best describes its purpose by placing the emphasis on the user. Standard D1 of CPA(UK)Ltd requires that 'There is an up-to-date user manual prepared in consultation with the service users'. In addition to the users handbook, there are a number of other opportunities for communication between clinician and laboratory. Request forms from clinicians and the reports issued by the laboratory are the main forms of written communication, but additionally there are a diverse range of meetings including clinico-pathological conferences and audit meetings (see Chapter 11) at which communication between clinicians and the laboratory can take place.

LABORATORY USERS HANDBOOK

Although the content of the users handbook is of prime importance, its presentation is equally important and careful thought should be given to its design, size and durability. The first question to consider is whether it should be in the form of a bound booklet or loose leaf. The pro's and con's are difficult. A booklet in an A5 presentation is commonly used as it fits well into the outside pocket of a doctor's white coat, but used in these circumstances it will need a laminated cover to give it durability. The advantage of a loose leaf format, whether it is in an A5 binder or in the increasingly popular *'Filofax'©* format, is that updated pages can be issued. However, because of the numbers of copies of the

Laboratory Users handbook that have to be issued, the process of update will not be easy to control. On balance the bound format is probably easier to control as new editions can be circulated with a letter requesting the recipients to destroy their previously issued edition and perhaps with a return slip requiring acknowledgement of receipt. Many accreditation systems require an annual revision of the users handbook but the term 'review' is more appropriate because it allows thought to be given to whether a revised version is necessary, without making it mandatory.

The content of the handbook will depend to some extent on who the user is likely to be, e.g. handbooks for laboratories which are not directly connected to a hospital may not have a description of blood collections on hospital wards, but may need to describe the arrangements for the dispatch and receipt of specimens sent by air. The model contents given in Figure 9.3 are based on a number of different guidelines and are not intended to include each subspeciality in pathology, but rather to point the way in relation to key issues. Details of the guidelines are to be found in Further Reading.

1.0 Contents

2.0 General Information

- Postal address
- Key personnel, their position and telephone, E mail and facsimile numbers
- Population served
- Laboratory hours including out of hours service

3.0 Use of the Laboratory

3.1 Requesting and collection of specimens

- Requesting procedures (routine, urgent and out of hours)
- Completing the request form
- Patient identification and specimen collection (for inpatient, outpatient or domicillary)
- Specimen labelling (including notification of infectious disease hazard)
- Specimen containers and where to get them

3.2 Transport to the laboratory

- Specimen delivery to the laboratory (including courier services and ward rounds)
- Portering schedules
- Use of pneumatic-tube delivery system if appropriate

3.3 Results including types and time of reporting

3.4 Tests requiring appointments

3.5 Information concerning clinics (e.g. anticoagulation)

3.6 Notification of the laboratory by clinicians of unexplained or clinically inconsistent results

3.7 Importance of the provision of clinical information to the laboratory

---

4.0 Departmental information

4.1 Biochemistry

- Tests provided on call
- Biochemical mini-profiles
- Information regarding dynamic function tests
- Therapeutic drug monitoring
- Storing specimens overnight
- Urine and faecal collections - special instructions
- Near patient testing

4.2 Haematology and Blood transfusion

- Tests provided on call
- Haematology mini-profiles
- Clotting studies
- Bone marrow examination
- *In vivo* investigations
- Blood group (antenatal and transfusion)
- Cross matching (routine and emergency)
- Use of blood products (clinical procedures)
- Transfusion reaction procedures

4.3 Histopathology (Anatomical Pathology)

- Surgical biopsies
- Frozen section bookings
- Requests for post-mortems
- Coroners autopsies

4.4 Cytopathology

- Special requirements for each type of specimen, e.g. Cervical smear

4.5 Microbiology

- Tests provided on call
- Antibiotic advice
- Hospital infection
- Blood culture - detailed method of collection
- Urine, faecal and seminal fluid - special instructions

5.0 Alphabetical tables of tests/procedures

These tables can be divided by discipline and should include:-

- Name of the test
- Specimen and container required
- Reference intervals (where appropriate)
- Special comments
- Turnaround time

Figure 9.3   Contents of pathology users handbook

REQUEST FORMS

In some countries the request form is called a requisition form. The majority of requests made by clinicians for tests and investigations are made using a request/requisition form. In some hospitals however, computer terminals are available in the wards or other situations which connect with the laboratory computer, either directly by a local area network, or through an order communications system enabling requests to be made on the laboratory computer. When such systems are in use the patient's identification details are normally obtained from the patient master index of the hospital patient management system (PMS) or from the laboratory computer's patient database which can in turn be refreshed periodically by information from the PMS. This obviates the problems of transcribing the doctors handwriting and, in the case of hospital inpatients, ties the patient identification to what is hopefully, but not always reliably, a unique hospital number. Further information on the management and operation of such systems is given in the section on computers in the laboratory.

Information	Reason

Patient's name
    unit number
    date of birth
    sex
	Identification and (age, sex) interpretation of results

Return address (e.g. ward, clinic, surgery; telephone/page number if urgent)	Delivery of report
Name of clinician (and telephone/ page number)	Liaison, Auditing, Billing
Clinical details (including drug treatment)	Justification of request Audit Interpretation Selection of appropriate tests Choice of analytical method (to avoid drug interference)
Test requested	Instruction to analyst
Sample(s) required	Instruction to phlebotomist
Date (and time if appropriate)	Identification Interpretation (with timed/sequential requests) Audit from Clinical Biochemistry, edited by Marshall WJ and Bangert SK Churchill Livingstone (1995)

Figure 9.4   Information required on a completed request form

The request form in pathology is the equivalent of a referral letter from one doctor to another and can be regarded as the first step in a consultation between the requesting doctor and the laboratory. In order for the laboratory to undertake its tasks properly, the request form must be designed in a way which makes it easy for the requesting doctor to provide necessary information. Information is required for a number of specific purposes which are outlined in Figure 9.4, knowledge of which is particularly important when training the staff who undertake the rather monotonous task of data acquisition.

There is a tendency in some laboratories to have a larger number of specialised request forms for particular situations. However, the fewer request forms that are presented to the requesting doctor the easier it is for the necessary information to be provided. Increasing numbers of laboratories have one request form for biochemistry, haematology and microbiology. An example of the general form used by St Elsewhere's Hospital Trust is given in Figure 9.5. Specialised forms should be restricted to areas such as requests for cervical cytology, blood transfusion, etc.

| **St Elsewhere's Hospital Trust - Pathology Laboratory** | **Telephone** | **(0800) 100200** |
| | **Facsimile** | **(0800) 300400** |

PATIENT NUMBER

LABORATORY ACCESSION NUMBER

SURNAME

REQUESTING DOCTOR   Signature
(please print name)

FORENAMES

Bleep number

ADDRESS

HOSPITAL   WARD/CLINIC

DATE & TIME OF COLLECTION

DATE OF BIRTH   SEX male/female

CONSULTANT/GENERAL PRACTITIONER
(Name and number)

CLINICAL DETAILS/DIAGNOSIS/THERAPY

BIOCHEMISTRY	HAEMATOLOGY	MICROBIOLOGY
☐ Renal profile ☐ Lipid profile	☐ Full blood count ☐ RA Latex	URINE ☐ MSU
☐ Liver profile ☐ Diabetic profile	☐ ESR ☐ Anti nuclear factor	☐ CSU
☐ Bone profile ☐ Fasting glucose	☐ B12 & folate ☐ Warfarin control (INR)	FAECES ☐ Culture
☐ Cardiac profile ☐ Random glucose	☐ Ferritin ☐ Coagulation screen	☐ Parasites
☐ Thyroid profile ☐ Pregnancy test	☐ IM screen ☐ Heparin control (APTT)	SPUTUM ☐ Routine
Please specify other items	Please specify other items	☐ AFB
		SWAB ☐ Cervical
		☐ HVS
		☐ Urethral
		Other from where CLOTTED BLOOD for... OTHER SPECIMEN for...

Figure 9.5   The general request form

The NCCLS produced a guideline on 'Development of Requisition Forms for Therapeutic Drug Monitoring (TDM) and/or Overdose Toxicology' and it gives a checklist of suggested data items on such specialised requisition forms (Figure 9.6).

In the above guideline the concept of a joint requisition/report form is discussed. It can be accomplished by having duplicate no carbon required (NCR) forms, or by photocopying the completed joint requisition/report form and sending out the photocopy. If one copy of the NCR form is returned to the requesting doctor, care must be taken that it is not contaminated with biological material during its transit through the laboratory. Photocopying, although time-consuming, obviates this problem. This concept may still have validity in a laboratory without computerisation, and has the advantage that the information provided, including the clinical reason for the request, is returned to the requesting doctor whether it is legible or not! Indeed the introduction of computers and the hugely escalating workload in many laboratories has made the availability of the 'reasons for a request' at time of reporting increasingly difficult to achieve.

The Patient

1. Identification[1,2]
   - Name
   - Address
   - Identification number or bar code

2. Weight

3. Age

4. Sex

5. Physiological factors[1]

6. Biological individuality

7. Drugs or other relevant substances (including food products) administered or consumed[1,2]

8. Primary disease or condition affecting the patient[1]

9. Intercurrent diseases affecting the patient

10. Other pertinent clinical information

Specimen information

1. Time of specimen collection [1,2]

2. Identifying specimens requiring immediate analysis

3. Requesting physician [1,2]

4. Location of the patient [2]

5. Type of specimen [1,2]

6. Analysis of interest or suspected drug [1,2]

[1] Essential information for therapeutic drug monitoring

[2] Essential information for overdose toxicology

adapted from 'Development of Requisition forms for Therapeutic Drug Monitoring and/or Overdose Toxicology' Approved guideline (1991) NCCLS Document T/DM1-A

Figure 9.6   Data items required for TDM or overdose toxicology requisition form

---

IDENTIFICATION, COLLECTION AND TRANSPORTATION

PATIENT IDENTIFICATION

The mechanism by which the specimen is associated with the patient and the request card is of utmost importance. When the association needs to be proven for legal purposes, then every step in operating process activities may have to be witnessed by a third party. This so called 'chain of custody' starts with the identification of the patient and continues through the whole operating process until the report is issued.

When a pathology specimen is collected from a patient, unique identification labels for the specimen are very rarely produced prior to or at the time of sampling. In some cases, however, there are computer systems (described earlier) which allow the request to be made to the laboratory via a remote terminal. These computer systems can prepare a phlebotomy work list with details of the patient's identity, their location in the hospital, and the investigations required. At the same time, a unique identification label(s) is produced for attaching to the specimen container(s). In this situation the person collecting the sample only has to positively identify the patient and collect the sample into the uniquely identified specimen container. Hospital inpatients normally wear identification bracelets which must be checked carefully before the specimen is collected. This process could be the first step in what is called 'positive specimen identification'. This is where the identification data, affixed to the specimen/container at source, remains with that specimen throughout analysis, is read electronically by laboratory analysers and computers and is printed on the final report without the need for manual transcript. In order to reduce transcription errors to a minimum each specimen has to be unequivocally identified as well as the patient who may well have more than one specimen in the laboratory at any one time.

More usually, however, a completed request card is received by the laboratory either with a specimen or in order to activate the phlebotomist or blood-taker into collecting the sample from the patient. It is important to ensure that certain minimum data is recorded on the specimen container and on the request card so that they can be unequivocally related. A minimum of information would be the name of the patient, date of birth, and the date of collection, preferably with some identification number relating to the hospital admission in the case of an inpatient.

SPECIMEN COLLECTION AND TRANSPORTATION

With many pathological specimens some of the most important sources of interference with the subsequent analysis can be associated with factors present at the time of sampling, and subsequent attempts to preserve or stabilise the specimens during transport or storage. There are a number of publications concerning the collection and transportation of pathological specimens and Further Reading gives some examples.

In addition to the collection and transportation of the sample, for certain biochemical and haematological tests it is important to standardise the preparation of the patient, e.g. fasting for sixteen hours for serum triglycerides, or be clear that the specimen has been collected at a specific time in relation to medication, e.g. therapeutic drug monitoring. Information concerning these issues should be included in the user handbook. Other clinical procedures provided by the laboratory and where possible prepared in conjunction with the appropriate clinicians, may include those for the collection of blood gases, conduct of glucose tolerance tests, and other dynamic function tests. If the procedure is novel or experimental then the approval of a local ethical committee must be sought.

In certain situations, particular care should be taken with regard to the adequacy of specimen collection, and in the case of cytopathology it is an important part of the receipt of the specimen that its adequacy should be determined.

SPECIMEN RECEPTION/DATA ACQUISITION

The arrangements in a pathology laboratory for specimen reception and data acquisition will vary according to how the laboratory is organised. Sometimes specimens go directly to the department concerned or there is a central area for the reception of all specimens, regardless of their ultimate destination. In the latter example a procedure should be written for specimen reception by such a central facility, and include the arrangements for subsequent despatch to the different disciplines/departments within pathology. If one department has special arrangements, such as the direct reception of specimens, e.g. biopsy specimens arriving from theatre for the histopathology department, such arrangements should be clearly delineated in the procedure.

The pathology department should encourage the request card and specimen container to be closely associated during transportation, by supplying specially designed polythene bags with separate compartments for specimen container(s) and request form. This is also good practice in relation to health and safety. During the process of initial sorting of specimens, care should be taken not to dissociate the relationship between the request form and the specimen. Only if unique identification was available for the sample container at the time of collection will the association be absolute. In most laboratories it is the practice to assign a label with an accession number (and sometimes other information, such as patient's name and tests required) to both the request form and the specimen container on arrival. Many laboratory computer systems allow the entry of patient identification data and the tests requested into the computer, which subsequently produces unique labels for the specimen container and request form. The procedure should ensure that such labels do not obscure any information already inscribed on the specimen container label or the request form, so that subsequent checks can be made to confirm the relationship between the request and the specimen.

It is not uncommon to find that the specimen reception and data acquisition functions are undertaken by junior members of the laboratory staff and a large part of the work is extremely repetitive. It is therefore important, firstly to arrange some variety in the duties of such personnel, secondly to ensure a training programme that not only teaches the task to be performed but also emphasises the critical importance of the work being undertaken, and finally to ensure a high level of supervision.

The term data is sometimes used interchangeably with information, but in this section it is used in a more restricted sense as being any series of observations, measurements or facts. This acquisition of data continues throughout the operating process until the reporting and interpretation stage, when it undergoes transformation into information or 'what the data conveys'. This is an important aspect of reporting because until a particular observation or measurement is interpreted by comparing the observation in the case of histopathology against what is known to occur in a particular pathological condition, or in the case of quantitative measurements referring to appropriate reference intervals, it lacks the value necessary to make it useful in patient care. Accurate acquisition of data and its presentation as information is not only important for this prime purpose of effective patient care but is also important for a range of management and business purposes, such as how many reagents to purchase for a particular analyser and where to send the bill! (Figure 9.1).

If the laboratory is not computerised then it will be necessary to maintain a record book in which details of the specimen(s) received and the identification of the patient are carefully recorded. Such records are often known as day books and are still maintained in some departments in addition to the computer record. With increasing demands upon pathology departments, however, this is only possible in those departments such as histopathology which receive relatively few requests, albeit the requests result in a large amount of work.

REFERRAL FOR SPECIALISED INVESTIGATIONS

In most pathology laboratories, however broad their repertoire of investigations, it will be necessary on certain occasions to refer tests to other laboratories. Possible reasons for referral might be for provision of a unique or unusual service, e.g. investigations or tests rarely performed by the sending laboratory, or for confirmation of initial unusual findings, for the provision of a backup service to the sending laboratory in the event of a planned or unforeseen interruption of service, or lastly referral of routine tests as part of a rationalisation of services between two or more laboratories. A laboratory should have a well documented and reliable system for tests referred and ensure that the results are returned and logged. The major concern in quality and accreditation systems about referral for specialised investigations is that the work should be undertaken in an approved or controlled facility.

The NCCLS have prepared a guideline on this topic entitled 'Selecting and Evaluating a Referral Laboratory' which seeks to identify objective criteria by which a laboratory could be judged. Most of the criteria are similar to those for any laboratory seeking to comply with the standards set by a recognised quality or accreditation system, but included in the checklist is the concept of the referring laboratory's reputation starting with the question 'Will the laboratory provide a list of key clients for you to contact?' One of the most important reasons for the referral of a specimen for a unique or unusual investigation is to benefit from the interpretative and clinical advice available in such centres, e.g. in the case of certain bone tumours, gut hormones or phage typing. Such knowledge is often built from personal contacts and it is not always possible to evaluate this objectively.

The matter of referral is mentioned specifically in CAP-LAP under Standard II Resources and Facilities: 'Tests may be performed by a reference laboratory or ancillary testing program if test results are provided in an effective manner and are of acceptable quality. Reference laboratories and ancillary testing programs must meet the needs of the patients and medical staff in timeliness, quality, and safety, and the referring laboratory's needs for compliance with accrediting and peer review agencies'. It continues 'If tests are to be referred to a reference laboratory, the laboratory director or consulting pathologist shall select the reference laboratory on the basis of objective evidence of acceptable quality. Except where special circumstances dictate otherwise, tests shall be referred to and analysed by laboratories that have been accredited by the College of American Pathologists or to the Joint Commission on Accreditation of Healthcare Organisations hospital laboratories. All referral laboratories must be CLIA certified for high complexity testing for all specialties/subspecialties for which they are providing testing.'

In EN 45001 there is a section 5.4.7 'Subcontracting' which requires that the testing laboratory shall normally perform the testing which they contract to undertake, but if they are to send any of the testing work to another laboratory, termed a subcontractor, then they must be sure and able to demonstrate that the subcontractor is competent with respect to the services provided. In ISO 9001:1994, paragraph 4.6 on Purchasing can be interpreted as a requirement for referral of tests and requires that 'The supplier (the laboratory) shall establish and maintain documented procedures to ensure that the purchased product conforms to specified requirements'. This might include requiring the laboratory to which the specimen is referred to provide evidence of participation and performance in external quality assessment schemes.

ANALYTICAL
The analytical phase of operating process activities is dealt with in Chapter 10.

POSTANALYTICAL

REPORTING AND INTERPRETATION
In this text the term 'reporting' includes both the content of the report and validation of the data and information which make up the content. When the report consists of sending out a photocopy of the request/requisition form then its design has to allow space in which to present the report, usually the design is such that the report is presented on the bottom half of the original request form. When the laboratory is computerised then a part of the report is composed of data acquired from the request form when it arrived with the specimen and in part from the subsequent measurements and observations made during the analytical process. As has been said in the section on specimen reception and data acquisition, it is how it is presented on the final report that determines its value as information.

The validation of data and information is an important part of the reporting procedure. Two types of validation are commonly described, technical validation and clinical validation. Later in this chapter a definition of validation is given in the context of computing (Figure 9.13). In this sense validation is 'the checking of data for correctness' and a computerised laboratory has a number of ways in which this can be performed. A report dependant on observations, such as the macroscopic and microscopic descriptions of tissue submitted for analysis, can be checked using a spell checker or, going back one stage, the report can in part be produced by automatic incorporation of phrases using brief mnemonics, such as 'spcon' equals 'The specimen consists of....'. The provision or ability to create a specialised or personal dictionary against which the spell checking is done is a normal part of present day computer systems.

Quantitative measurements can be subjected to checks which can activate different responses. If a haemoglobin or serum potassium result is outside one set of limits it can be flagged prior to technical validation and subsequent reporting as incompatible with life, or in other words a 'nonsense report'. Results can also be flagged during the reporting process as a critical value requiring immediate action such as telephoning the result, or alternatively it can be flagged on the report as outside appropriate reference intervals. These technical validation checks can be done without a computerised system but, as the volume of data produced per week by even a small laboratory is quite large, there are clearly limitations on what can be achieved.

The international definition of validation in relation to quality (ISO 8402:1994) 'confirmation by examination and provision of objective evidence that the particular requirements for a specific intended use are fulfilled' relate better to clinical validation. The process of clinical or medical validation, often called 'signing out' of reports, is where a senior member of the medical or scientific staff validates the report by scrutinising individual results for internal consistency or against clinical information provided on the request form. Where technical validation ends and clinical validation begins is not entirely clear. Some methods described under technical validation, such as a result being in a critical area, can be used to select particular results for the further process of clinical validation. The validation by scrutiny for internal consistency can be achieved using rule-based algorithms which can decide that 'normally' a high result for one analyte is incompatible with a low result for a second analyte, and flag that situation for attention. Logically the final clinical validation, albeit mainly retrospective, is the involvement of the laboratory in the activity of clinical audit (see Chapter 11).

A number of standards in quality and accreditation systems place great importance on the quality of reporting and the interpretation of results. Clearly, in certain disciplines the interpretation of the findings of an investigation *per se*, rather than in relation to a particular clinical setting, are a major part of the report and this is discussed further in the next chapter. Standard 2 of the NPAAC Standards for Pathology Laboratories give a clear indication of the requirement for the consultative aspect of a laboratory's work, and in particular the evaluation and interpretation of results (Figure 9.7).

STANDARD 2 - CONSULTATION

LABORATORIES SHALL HAVE STAFF WHO CAN ADVISE CLINICIANS ON THE EVALUA-
TION AND INTERPRETATION OF RESULTS OF LABORATORY EXAMINATIONS AND THE
PRECISION AND ACCURACY OF METHODS EMPLOYED IN THE LABORATORY

Commentary

An essential part of the laboratory activity is the provision of the consultative service to the clinician. The consulting service should be readily available and the clinician should be able to obtain authoritative advice from the laboratory on:

   (i)   the precision and accuracy of methods used in the laboratory;

  (ii) the statistical significance of results and their relation to reference ranges;

(iii) the scientific basis and the clinical significance of the results;

 (iv) the suitability of the requested procedure to solve the clinical problem in question; and

  (v) further procedures which may be helpful.

NPAAC Standards for Pathology Laboratories (1986)

Figure 9.7   NPAAC Standard 2 Consultation and commentary

In Section 5.4.3 of EN 45001:1989 it states 'The work carried out by the testing laboratory shall be covered by a report which accurately, clearly and unambiguously presents the test results and all other relevant information'. It goes on to say 'Each test report shall include at least the following information' and a comprehensive list is shown in Figure 9.8. However, later in that section it says 'A test report shall not include any advice or recommendation arising from the test results'. This stipulation would at first sight seem to be an alien concept in relation to pathology reporting unless it can be interpreted as meaning that in a test report 'advice and recommendations arising from the test results' should be clearly distinguished from the test results themselves.

Each test report shall include at least the following information:

a) Name and address of testing laboratory and location where the test was carried out when different from the address of the testing laboratory;

b) Unique identification of report (such as serial number) and of each page, and total number of pages of the report;

c) Name and address of client;

d) Description and identification of the test item;

e) Date of receipt of test item and date(s) of performance of test;

f) Identification of the test specification or description of the method or procedure;

g) Description of sampling procedure, where relevant;

h) Any deviations, additions to or exclusions from the test specification, and any other information relevant to a specific test;

i) Identification of any non-standard test method or procedure utilised;

j) Measurements, examinations and derived results, supported by tables, graphs, sketches and photographs as appropriate, and any failures identified;

k) A statement on measurement uncertainty (where relevant);

l) A signature and title or any equivalent marking of person(s) accepting technical responsibility for the test report and date of issue;

m) A statement to the effect that the test results relate only to the items tested;

n) A statement that the report shall not be reproduced except in full without the written approval of the testing laboratory.

EN 45001:1989 5.4.3 Test reports

Figure 9.8   EN 45001:1989 Content of the report

REQUIREMENTS FOR OPERATING PROCESS ACTIVITIES

Whereas the requirements of different quality and accreditation systems for the preanalytical, analytical and postanalytical phases of operating process activities are easy to distinguish for EN 45001:1989, CAP-LAP, and CPA(UK)Ltd, they are more difficult for ISO 9001:1994 and OECD-GLP. This difficulty stems from the origins of the systems and the different terms used for similar topics. A brief explanation may facilitate the identification of requirements in this area. As ISO 9001:1994 is a quality system intended for use by any organisation wishing to ensure the quality of its product(s), it is necessary to define the term product. Product is defined in the standard as the 'result of any activities or processes' and can include a service, hardware, processed material, software or a combination thereof. It can be tangible (e.g. assemblies or processed material) or intangible (e.g. knowledge or concepts), or a combination thereof. In the context of pathology, the main products are the reports of investigations carried out on biological specimens and the advice given on the report itself, or the consultation with the clinician from whose patient the original sample was obtained concerning the findings in the report. Figure 9.9 interprets the ISO terminology in terms of the activities of a pathology laboratory and should be used in conjunction with Figure 9.10 which interprets the clauses of ISO 9001:1994 associated with the operating process (see Figure 3.5).

Terms and definitions from ISO 8402 - 1994 (used in ISO 9001:1994)		Interpretation for the Pathology Laboratory
• customer	recipient of a product provided by a supplier	the **doctor** requesting investigation of a pathological specimen and recipient of the pathology report or in some circumstances the patient
• purchaser	customer in a contractual relationship	a **health organisation** purchasing on behalf of the doctor
• supplier	organisation that provides a product to a customer	the **pathology laboratory**
• subcontractor	organisation that provides a product to a supplier	**supplier of products or services** to the pathology laboratory, includes referred tests
• product	the result of activities or processes (see text for fuller description)	e.g. **the pathology report**
• service	result generated by activities at the interface between the supplier and the customer and by the supplier internally to meet the customer needs	e.g. **the consultation** between the clinician and the laboratory in connection with the pathology report

Figure 9.9   Interpretation of ISO terminology for the pathology laboratory

THE OPERATING PROCESS	INTERPRETATION OF ISO 9001:1994 FOR STEPS IN OPERATING PROCESS ACTIVITIES (*refer also to Figure 9.1*)
SALES AND MARKETING	**1. Doctor/patient relationship** **2. Request form completed**
4.3 Contract review	Clause 4.3 describes the review of the contracts between purchaser and supplier/provider. In some settings the doctor who requests investigations can be regarded as the purchaser and even if some other agency purchases on their behalf they should together with laboratory personnel define the requirements they have of the laboratory services. These deliberations may be reflected in a formal contract or informally in a Users Handbook or both.
DESIGN	
4.4 Design control	Clause 4.4 forms a part of ISO 9001:1994 but is only applicable if the laboratory is providing services which require the substantial development of new methods in the course of delivering the product (e.g. test result)
	3. Specimen collection **4. Specimen and request form transportation** **5. Specimen and request form reception** **6. Data acquisition from specimen and request form** **7. Specimen preparation** **8. Specimen analysis**
SHOPFLOOR *4.7 Control of customer-supplied products* *4.10 Inspection & testing* *4.9 Process control* *4.12 Inspection & test status* *4.13 Control of non conforming products*	Clause 4.7 concerns the procedures for the verification of receipt and storage of customer (doctor) supplied products (pathological specimens) together with notification to the customer of inadequacies in the specimens supplied. Clause 4.10 requires the proper inspection and control of all incoming products, pathological specimens and all reagents, consumables etc. required in all phases of the analytical process. Clause 4.9 concerns the procedures (operating process activity) required for achievement of a quality product (e.g. the laboratory report). Clauses 12 and 13 concern inspection and test status of the product (the results of analysis) to indicate conformance or non conformance, and the steps to take in respect of non conformance (quality control).
	9. Reporting of results including interpretation and recommendations **10. Transmission of results**
DISTRIBUTION *4.15 Handling, storage, packaging, preservation & delivery*	Clause 4.15 concerns requirements for the delivery of the product (issuing of reports).
	11. Receipt of reports by clinician and consultation as appropriate
AFTER SALES *4.19 Servicing*	Clause 4.19 equates with the servicing of the product and can be interpreted as the consultation that may or not occur with the clinician with respect to a particular issued report.

Figure 9.10   ISO 9001:1994 in terms of the steps in operating process activities

The terms used in OECD-GLP also need interpretation to understand their equivalence in pathology laboratory terms. Figure 9.11 describes the terms used, and arranges them approximately in order of operating process activity. A test system is defined as 'any animal, plant, microbial, as well as other cellular, subcellular, chemical, or physical system or combination thereof used in the study'. If investigations are being carried out on patients in a clinical trial, the test system would be the patient and the test substance the drug under trial. Specimens collected from the test system are equivalent to specimens collected from patients, and the final report in GLP is equivalent to the report sent out from a pathology laboratory.

Terms and definitions	from OECD-GLP	Interpretation for the Pathology Laboratory
• **sponsor**	person(s) or entity who commissions and/or supports a study	the **doctor** requesting investigation of a pathological specimen and recipient of the pathology report
• **study**	an experiment or set of experiments in which a test substance is examined to obtain data on its properties and/or its safety with respect to human health and the environment	the **investigations** required by a doctor investigating a patient's condition(s) *(see Figure 9.2 Reasons for ordering laboratory tests)* and defined on the **request form**
• **test substance**	a chemical substance or a mixture which is under investigation	the patient's **condition** which is under investigation (in a clinical trial this could be the drug under investigation)
• **test system**	any animal, plant, microbial, as well as other cellular, subcellular, chemical or physical system or thereof used in the study	the **patient**
• **specimens**	any material derived from the test system for examination, analysis or storage	Specimens collected from the patient and submitted for analysis
• **study plan**	a document which defines the entire scope of the study	all the **procedures** to be used by the doctor/ laboratory to investigate the patient's condition, including the analytical procedures used
• **raw data**	all original laboratory records and documentation, or verified copies thereof, which are the result of the original observations and activities in the study	**raw data** has the same meaning
• **final report**	a document describing the outcome of the study	e.g. **the pathology report** including any interpretation and consultation

Figure 9.11   Interpretation of OECD-GLP terminology for the pathology laboratory

REQUIREMENTS FOR PRE AND POSTANALYTICAL PHASES OF OPERATING PROCESS ACTIVITIES

The requirements for the preanalytical and postanalytical phases of operating process activities in quality and accreditation systems are shown in Figure 9.12, and for the analytical phase in Figure 10.6 of the next chapter.

System	Preanalytical and postanalytical phases of operating process activities
ISO 9001:1994	*(see Figure 9.9 and 9.10 for further information)*
EN 45001:1989	**5. Technical competence** **5.4 Working procedures** *5.4.5 Handling of test samples or items* 'A system for identifying the samples or items to be tested or calibrated shall be applied, either through documents or through marking, to ensure that there can be no confusion regarding the identity of the samples or items and the results of the measurements made…' There shall be clear rules for the receipt, retention and disposal of samples or items. *5.4.3 Test reports* The work carried out by the testing laboratory shall be recovered by a report which accurately, clearly and unambiguously presents the test results and all other relevant information. *(further details are shown in Figure 9.8)*
OECD - GLP	**7. Standard Operating Procedures** **7.1 General** *The nearest equivalent to a request procedure is in section :-* **8.Performance of the Study** *which requires that a study should be formulated in a* **study plan** *The nearest equivalent to a report is in section :-* **9.Reporting of Study Results** *which requires the preparation of a* **final report**. *(see Figure 9.11 for further information)*
CAP - LAP	**Standard IV Quality control** in the interpretation of the standard it says:- 'Written instructions shall be available that provide, in detail, the methods for procuring, transporting, and processing appropriate specimens. There shall be a written description of the system for the timely reporting of patient data to the physician and of the safeguards taken to ensure that such data is correct'.
CPA(UK)Ltd	**D Policies and procedures** **D1** There is an up to date user manual. **D2** Request forms for laboratory investigations and specimen labels include provision for unique patient identification and adequate supporting information. **D3** Reports of laboratory results are validated prior to despatch, are timely, and include unique patient identity, date of testing/reporting, and name and location of requesting clinician. **D4** Interpretative reports are accurate, comprehensive and clinically relevant.

	D5 There are written procedures relating to specimen collection, handling and disposal.
	D9 There is a written procedure for the reporting of results of each test.
	D10 There is a written procedure for oral transmission of results.

Figure 9.12 Requirements for pre and postanalytical phases of operating process activities

COMPUTERS IN THE LABORATORY

DEFINITIONS

Before starting this section on computers it may be useful to set out some of the definitions of the fundamental terms used in computing (Figure 9.13).

Computer: A device consisting of one or more associated processing units and peripheral units that is controlled by internally stored programmes which can perform arithmetic calculations and other logical operations without outside intervention.

Data*: A representation of facts, concepts, or instructions in a formalised manner suitable for communication, interpretation, or processing by humans or by automatic means.

Data-processing: The capture, storage, and processing of data to transform it into information more suitable for decision making.

File (computer)*: A set of related records treated as a unit.

Hardware*: Physical equipment in contrast to software.

Interface*: A shared boundary between two functional units defined by functional characteristics, common physical interconnection characteristics or signal characteristics, as appropriate. The concept involves the specification of the connection of two devices having different functions.

Program: A set of instructions for the computer to follow.

Record: A group of related data elements treated as a unit.

Software: Programs, procedures, rules and any associated documentation pertaining to the operation of a computer system.

Validation (Computer): The checking of data for correctness, or compliance with applicable (of data processing) standards, rules and conventions. In the context of equipment rather than data, validation involves checking for correct performance etc.

Based on ISO 2382-1:1984 marked * and from Accreditation for Chemical Laboratories
EURACHEM Guidance document No 1 /WELAC Guidance Document No. WGD 2.

Figure 9.13 Definitions of fundamental terms used in computing

In Chapter 4, Figure 4.1 showed the hierarchy of documents with the form at the bottom of the pyramid, and indicating that when data was entered onto the form it became a record. Figure 9.14 shows different approaches to data collection. A hard copy multi-entry form is shown with headings A-F which indicate where to enter data, (A = Hospital number, B = Patients name, etc.). When the data (a_1 b_1 etc.) is entered, this document is then called a record. Similarly, with the hard copy single entry forms, when they have data entered they become records. When this data is entered into the computer it goes into a computer file which is an electronic record. Such a file will have headings but in this environment they are called 'fields', and also the word 'record' is used not to refer to the whole file but in a more specific sense to 'a group of related data elements treated as a unit' for example a_2, b_2, c_2, d_2, e_2, and f_2.

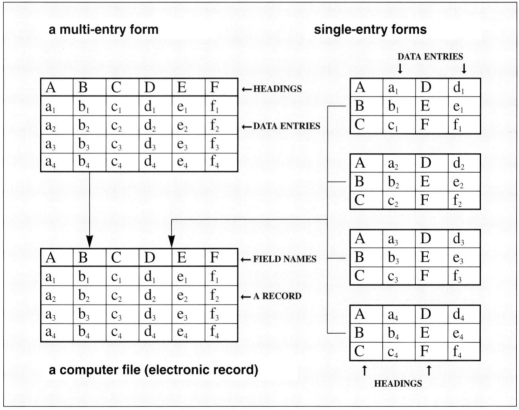

Figure 9.14 Forms, records, fields and files

The other term commonly in use is 'database' which has been described as 'any file which might sound more important if called a database'*. Finally, another important term is

*The Penguin Dictionary of Microprocessors, Anthony Chandor, (1981)

'relational database' because the design of a laboratory computer system is often based on such a structure. It can be defined as 'a database using a relational data model and the data is stored in the form of several two dimensional tables or flat files. The tables embody different ideas about the data but contain overlapping information'. For example, one file might store some serum amylase results against a mnemonic for serum amylase (SAMY) and the accession number given to that particular request. Another file might hold the accession number and patient demographic information such as date of birth (age), and sex, and a third file the mnemonic for serum amylase, and information about the units used for reporting and reference intervals for age and sex. All these separate files, and more, would be used to print a report.

USE OF COMPUTERS

Computers are used very extensively in many pathology laboratories. Examples of such uses are shown in Figure 9.15. This section will concentrate on the principle aspects of the management of a main laboratory computer. However, much of what is said will apply to other computer systems in the pathology laboratory. Typically such a computer will not only capture, process, report and store data concerning the identification of patients and specimen analysis, but will also be able to communicate the results back to the requesting doctor. Automated laboratory equipment is controlled by computers, and the software which comes with these computers can prove more of a problem in the early evaluation than do mechanical functions of the equipment. The use of personal computers in the laboratory is now extensive and includes the creation and management of laboratory documentation, and the use of costing and financial management programmes.

- Communication between the requester and the laboratory
- Acquisition, processing, reporting and storage of data
- Quality control and assessment data evaluation and presentation
- Operation and control of automated equipment
- Direct/indirect capture of data from automated equipment
- Matching of sample and library data
- Performance of statistical functions
- Creation and management of laboratory documentation
- Monitoring and control of inventories
- Stock control of reagents, consumables and standard material
- Costing and financial management programmes

Figure 9.15   Uses of computers in the pathology laboratory

ORGANISATION AND MANAGEMENT

In the pathology laboratory of St Elsewhere's Hospital Trust the main day to day responsibility for running the Pathology Laboratory computer (ABC-3500) is carried by the Computer Manager (see Figure 6.5 for the job description) who reports to the Business Manager. The Director of the laboratory has overall responsibility for the management arrangements but delegates this responsibility to a suitably experienced colleague who acts as chairman of the Laboratory Computer Working Group. The Computer Manager acts as secretary to the working group, and other members include the discipline specific database co-ordinators and representatives of other users, e.g. clerical staff. The discipline database co-ordinators are appropriately trained laboratory staff who work closely with the Computer Manager to ensure that changes in hardware, software and database information are carried out in a structured, documented and reliable fashion. Although one of the main functions of the Laboratory Computer Working Group is the management of the Pathology Laboratory Computer, it also co-ordinates strategies regarding the purchase and maintenance of personal computers and their applications software.

FACILITIES AND EQUIPMENT

In some countries it is mandatory that any computer system which holds information concerning individual patients or members of staff, must be registered under data protection legislation (for further discussion see under Security).

For each application there should be documentation fully describing:

* The name of the application software or identification code and a detailed and clear description of the purpose of the application.

* The hardware (with model numbers) on which the application software operates.

* The operating system and other system software (e.g. tools) used in conjunction with the application.

* The application programming language(s) and/or database tools used.

* The major functions performed by the application.

* An overview of the type and flow of data/data design associated with the application.

* File structures, error and alarm messages, and algorithms associated with the application.

* The application software components with version numbers.

* Configuration and communication links among application modules and to equipment and other systems.

from Section 8 Documentation in 'The application of the principles of GLP to computerised systems' Environmental Monograph No 116 OECD Paris 1995

Figure 9.16 OECD-GLP requirements for application description

Under this legislation it is not only important that the computer facilities should be registered, but also that procedures are in place to enable information regarding individuals to be readily accessible upon request. The computer hardware, like any other piece of equipment in the laboratory, should be subject to the procedure for management of equipment described in Chapter 7, including a record in the equipment inventory (Figure 7.15).

In addition, however, certain quality and accreditation systems require that details of applications running on the hardware should be kept. This is best done as a record on a separate form in a manual system or as a separate file in a relational database linked to the main file in the equipment inventory system through a unique number in both files. Figure 9.16 indicates suggested contents for such a form.

Computer installations will normally produce a large amount of heat and therefore will require some form of air-conditioning or, to be environmentally friendly, some system for re-utilising the heat produced (see item 2 in Figure 7.10).

MAINTENANCE AND DISASTER RECOVERY

The increasing dependence of laboratories on the reliability of computer installations makes the maintenance of these pieces of equipment very important. It is important to have a preventative maintenance contract which not only covers the maintenance of the hardware of the computer, but also covers the maintenance of the integrity of the operating system and laboratory applications software. A further development of this arrangement is a 'facilities management' system where the computer is provided and run by a commercial concern for an annual fee. The actual installation can be in the laboratory or a remote site. Even with commercially available systems, a laboratory can become over-dependent on one person to maintain the system. It is not unusual to find a laboratory being run on 'home grown' computer programmes written by one person. It is crucial that these systems are properly documented and that other staff are trained to cope with emergency breakdowns on such systems.

Procedures need to be in place which deal with the partial or total failure of any computer system. When a piece of automated equipment is controlled by a computer, this can cause particular problems if the computer fails as it is impossible to decontaminate the equipment without a functioning computer. For this reason a clause is included in the form for Equipment Servicing Declaration of Decontamination Status and Authorisation to Work (see Figure 7.16). Section C states 'This equipment/item has not been decontaminated and the nature and risk of the safety precautions to be adopted are…' Plans need to be made that will not only result in the recovery of the computerised system but include mechanisms for ensuring the integrity of the data recovered. Should the 'down time' be extensive, then plans need to be well-documented for the continuing provision of service, particularly in relation to work done on emergency specimens.

DATA MANAGEMENT

In certain accreditation systems the maintenance of raw data is regarded as essential. In OECD-GLP it is defined as being 'all the original laboratory records and documentation or verified copies thereof, which are the result of the original observations and activities and the activities in the study', and will include all data on computer files whether the entry is indirect or directly through an instrument interface. It is important to be able to identify the audit trail for such data, and the laboratory computer should have the ability to associate all changes to data with the persons making those changes. This is often assured by access security being arranged in such a way that changes are logged in terms of timed and dated electronic signatures. In order to validate raw data or reconstruct an analytical pathway, it may be necessary to also retain supporting information which may not be held on the computer, such as maintenance and calibration records.

SECURITY

It is important that security measures are in place to restrict access to any computer equipment. This often means that the security of the whole pathology laboratory should be maintained, as not all equipment will be found in a particular 'computer room'. Logical security requires that the user needs to enter a unique electronic signature or password which not only allows the user to use the computer, but also defines the level of access. The user's level of access will relate to the type of responsibility and tasks they have to perform. For example, a member of the laboratory staff who is responsible for entering information from request forms and specimen labels will only require the level of access to enable them to perform these particular functions. In general, an individual's access should be restricted to those functions which it is necessary for them to perform.

It is also important to appreciate that data or software which comes to the laboratory on any form of electronic medium should be checked for viruses before it is introduced into the system. This is an increasing problem for all computers, and they should be provided with the most recent virus detection programmes. Failure to do this can lead to the irretrievable loss of data. It is important, not only that people are given electronic signatures, but that they understand the importance of the maintenance of data integrity on the system, and this should be part of their training.

The procedure for preparing backup copies of all the software should be clearly delineated. This will include not only back-up copies of the data files, but also of the operating and applications software. Some hospital computer systems include laboratory modules, and the computing facility of the laboratory may then be situated and maintained outside the pathology laboratory. It is important to ensure under these circumstances that the procedure for the management of the laboratory computer encompasses a clear description of these arrangements, and how they might affect the integrity of data.

The Council of the European Union have recently published a new draft directive on 'the protection of individuals with regard to the processing of personal data and on the free movement of such data' and in the UK the British Medical Association have produced some interim guidelines on clinical system security. In addition they have commissioned the development of a clinical information security policy which sets out nine principles of data security (Figure 9.17), designed to uphold the principle of patient consent and to be independent of specific equipment.

---

(1) **Access control** - Each identifiable clinical record shall be marked with an access control list naming the people or groups of people who may read it and append data to it. The system shall prevent anyone not on the list from accessing the record in any way.

(2) **Record opening** - A clinician may open a record with herself and the patient on the access control list. When a patient has been referred she may open a record with herself, the patient, and the referring clinician(s) on the access control list.

(3) **Control** - One of the clinicians on the access control list must be marked as being responsible. Only she may change the access control list and she may add only other health care professionals to it.

(4) **Consent and notification** - The responsible clinician must notify the patient of the names of his record's access control list when it is opened, of all subsequent additions, and whenever responsibility is transferred. His consent must also be obtained, except in emergency or in the case of statutory exemptions.

(5) **Persistence** - No one shall have the ability to delete clinical information until the appropriate time has expired.

(6) **Attribution** - All accesses to clinical records shall be marked on the record with the name of the person accessing the record as well as the date and time. An audit trail must be kept of all deletions.

(7) **Information flow** - Information derived from record A may be appended to record B if and only if B's access control list is contained in A's.

(8) **Aggregation control** - Effective measures should exist to prevent the aggregation of personal health information. In particular, patients must receive special notification if any person whom it is proposed to add to their access control list already has access to personal health information on a large number of people.

(9) **Trusted computing base** - Computer systems that handle personal health information shall have a subsystem that enforces the above principles in an effective way. Its effectiveness shall be evaluated by independent experts.

Anderson R, Clinical system security: interim guidelines
BMJ 1996;312:109-11

Figure 9.17 Nine principles of data security

VALIDATION

As with any piece of equipment, procedures should be in place governing the acceptance of equipment and its validation in relation to the original memorandum of specification. In certain cases it may be important to be able to carry out a retrospective evaluation of the computer installation. Figure 9.13 gives a formal definition of computer validation and Figure 9.18 translates this into a working definition. This process is part of what is termed 'change control' described below.

Computer validation

Computers whatever their type, suffer from the 'black-box' syndrome: an input is made at one end, an answer is produced at the other. Because what happens inside cannot be seen, it must be assumed that the box is functioning correctly. For the purposes of validation it is usually acceptable to assume correct operation if the computer produces expected answers when input with well-characterised parameters.

The degree of validation necessary depends on the exact use of the computer. For each computer, the proposed use should be defined so that the degree of validation necessary may be established.

from Accreditation for Chemical Laboratories
EURACHEM Guidance document No.1 /WELAC Guidance Document No. WGD 2

Figure 9.18 Definition of computer validation

An important part of computer management is the proper application of a change control mechanism where there is formal approval and documentation of any change to a computerised system. The computer manager should be given the primary responsibility of maintaining such records, and it is important that the computer manager works in close conjunction with people appointed as departmental database co-ordinators. This topic of change control has been usefully termed 'configuration management' and is defined as 'a set of procedures that when followed, ensure adequate control, visibility and security of the version number, issue, and any changes made to hardware programme source codes, executable object codes, firmware, data, and electronic representation of documents. The procedures require any modifications made, as well as the personnel making them, to be authorised. The details of such changes shall be correctly recorded, together with details and results of tests carried out to validate the modified computer system' (see Further Reading). It may be necessary to establish a separate procedure for this process or include it in a Procedure for the Management of Computers (see Figure 9.20).

DOCUMENTATION AND RECORDS

Figure 9.19 shows the range of documentation associated with the management and day-to-day operation of the Pathology Laboratory Computer ABC-3500. In management terms it is subject to two management procedures, firstly the procedure for management of equipment (see Figure 7.19) and associated forms (see Figure 7.17) and secondly, the procedure for management of laboratory computers (Figure 9.20), and associated forms for applications description, and change control. Laboratory procedures will also be required for the day-to-day use of the computer and these should be documented within the management procedure. Any changes in these procedures should be subject to authorisation by the computer manager who should also be responsible for initiating training in any new procedures.

The (laboratory) procedure/working instructions for the Pathology Laboratory Computer ABC-3500 [LP 000 002], together with some of the content of the manufacturers user manuals, are used for routine operations of the computer. However, manufacturers user manuals for main pathology computers are not generally user-friendly and a great deal of work is often necessary in order to produce a good practical procedure that can be understood by all the laboratory staff who have cause to use the computer.

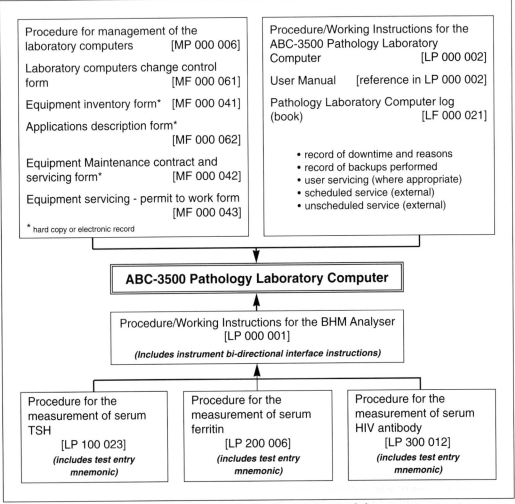

Figure 9.19 Documentation and records for the ABC-3500 laboratory computer

The pathology laboratory computer will often be interfaced to a number of different laboratory analysers and Figure 9.19 indicates that instructions regarding the instrument bi-directional interface for the BHM Analyser are given in the laboratory procedure/working instructions [LP 000 001]. Finally, laboratory procedures for the different analyses will contain details of the mnemonic required to order a particular test. A table of such mnemonics might also form part of the procedure for the ABC-3500 computer itself and be available to each VDU used for inputting patient data and test requests.

ARCHIVES

Even with large computers, there is a practical limitation on the amount of data that can be stored. Theoretically there should be no such limitation, and all data should be instantly available. However, it is often uneconomic to maintain all data on the system. It is therefore necessary to delineate an archiving policy and determine which particular item in a record will trigger an archive. In pathology laboratory systems the archiving is often triggered by a certain period of inactivity on the patient's record, such that if a patient has not presented for further work in the laboratory for six months their records are then archived.

It is important that any system of archiving has a system of indexing which will enable relatively rapid retrieval. Archiving is done on some form of electronic media, and the storage of these disks or tapes should be subject to proper conditions of environmental control so that they cannot suffer damage and loss. It may be necessary to dispose of archive material, but this must not be done without authorisation at the level of the Director of Pathology or the head of department. Arrangements will need to be made for short-term and long-term access to archived material. Short-term access does not normally constitute a problem as a disk or tape can be reloaded on the system and searched in a reasonably convenient manner. However, if it is intended that there should be long-term storage of archived material, it may be that the computer system has changed both in terms of hardware and software. In this situation thought will be needed about long-term storage of the data and of the operating and applications software to enable retrieval of the data should a suitable computer platform still be available. Archived material and at least one copy of current backup material should be stored in a secure location, separate from the computer room and preferably separate from the laboratory.

TRAINING

All staff who have to use the computer, for whatever task, should be given adequate training. If they have access to the management programmes of the equipment it is often better if the original supplier trains them. With regard to software for personal computers, there are a number of companies who will arrange the training of staff on an off-site or on-site basis. Although the initial expenditure may seem large, it is worthwhile in the long-term to ensure that training is done properly, because many software packages are in practice only utilised to some 20% of their capacity.

PROCEDURE FOR THE MANAGEMENT OF THE LABORATORY COMPUTER

The content of a procedure for the management of the laboratory computer is shown in Figure 9.20.

Content of the procedure (references to Figures in brackets)	
1.0 Purpose and scope	6.5 Security
2.0 Responsibilities	6.5.1 Physical security
3.0 References	6.5.2 Logical security
4.0 Definitions	6.5.3 Control of external data and software
5.0 Documents	6.5.4 Data integrity
6.0 Actions and Methods	6.5.5 Backup
6.1 Organisation and management	6.6 Validation
6.1.1 Laboratory Computer Working Group	6.6.1 Acceptance
6.1.2 Director of Pathology	6.6.2 Retrospective evaluation
6.1.3 Laboratory staff	6.6.3 Change control
6.1.4 Computer manager *(Figure 6.5 Job description)*	6.7 Documentation
6.1.5 Departmental database	6.7.1 Application description (Figure 9.15)
6.2 Facilities and equipment	6.7.2 Procedures
6.2.1 Environmental control	6.7.3 Forms and records
6.2.2 Hardware inventory *(Figure 7.15 Equipment inventory)*	6.8 Archives
6.2.3 Communications inventory	6.8.1 Archiving
6.2.4 Software inventory including licences *(see Section 6.7.1)*	6.8.2 Archive indexing
	6.8.3 Archive storage (including environmental control)
6.2.5 Data protection registration	6.8.4 Archive disposal
6.3 Maintenance and disaster recovery	6.8.5 Short term and long term access
6.3.1 Maintenance - contracts for prevention and fault repair	6.9 Training
6.3.2 System disaster recovery plan	6.10 Audit
6.3.3 Contingency plan	
6.4 Data management	
6.4.1 Definition of raw data	
6.4.2 Identification of audit trails	*based upon 'The application of the principles of GLP to*
6.4.3 Retention of supporting information (maintenance and calibration records)	*computerised systems' Environmental Monograph No.116 OECD Paris 1995*

Figure 9.20 Contents of a procedure for management of laboratory computers

REQUIREMENTS FOR MANAGEMENT OF COMPUTERS

The requirements for management and operation of computers in the different quality and accreditation schemes are shown in Figure 9.21.

System	Management of computers
ISO 9001:1994	**4. Quality system requirements** No specific reference to computer management but footnotes in certain sections say records may be in the form of any type of media, such as hard copy or electronic media which implies that all the appropriate sections will apply to data handling by computers.
EN 45001:1989	**5. Technical competence** **5.4 Working procedures** *5.4.1 Test methods and procedures* …Where results are derived by electronic data processing techniques, the reliability and stability of the system shall be such that the accuracy of the results is not affected. The system shall be able to detect malfunctions during programme execution and take appropriate action.
OECD - GLP	**3. Facilities** *No specific reference to computers but see Further Reading, 'The application of the principles of GLP to computerised systems' Environmental Monograph No.116 OECD Paris 1995, and Figure 9.16.*
CAP - LAP	**Standard II Resources and facilities** The pathology service shall have sufficient and appropriate space, equipment, facilities…In addition, the pathology service shall have effective methods for communication to ensure prompt and reliable reporting. There shall be appropriate record storage and retrieval. (Further specific questions and commentary are found in the CAP-LAP Inspection checklist Laboratory General Section I)
CPA(UK)Ltd	**Facilities and equipment** **C6.** There are appropriate and adequate data storage, retrieval and communication facilities. Guidelines: 1. There should be logbooks, filing systems or computerised data processing which are acceptable, in particular with relation to patient confidentiality. 2. All systems, including any manual backup, are tried, tested and functional. 3. Computer systems must be robust and reliable, data properly backed up in secure storage safe from fire. 4. There must be adequate provision of telephones, fax machines, and intercoms. 5. Departments should comply with the Data Protection Act 1984 and the laboratory should follow current guidelines related to data retention. 6. Where appropriate and requested, the laboratory data systems and data sets should conform to the requirements of the local cancer registry.

Figure 9.21 Requirements for management of computers

FURTHER READING

PRE AND POSTANALYTICAL PHASES OF OPERATING PROCESS ACTIVITIES

Blood Gas Preanalytical Considerations: Specimen Collection, Calibration, and Controls; Approved Guideline 1993, NCCLS Document C27-A.

Blood Collection on Filter Paper for Neonatal Screening Programs - Second Edition; Approved Standard 1992, NCCLS Document LA4-A2.

Collection, Transport and Processing of Blood Specimens for Coagulation Testing and Performance of Coagulation Assays - Second Edition; Approved Guideline 1991, NCCLS Document H21-A2.

Development of Requisition Forms for Therapeutic Drug Monitoring and/or Overdose Toxicology; Approved Guideline 1991, NCCLS Document T/DM1-A.

Devices for Collection of Skin Puncture Blood Specimens - Second Edition; Approved Guideline 1990, NCCLS Document H14-A2.

Evacuated Tubes for Blood Specimen Collection - Third Edition; Approved Standard 1991, NCCLS Document H1-A3.

Fine-Needle Aspiration Biopsy (FNAB) Techniques; Proposed Guideline 1994, NCCLS Document GP20-P.

How to Define, Determine, and Utilize Reference Intervals in the Clinical Laboratory; Approved Guideline 1995, NCCLS Document C28-A.

Percutaneous Collection of Arterial Blood for Laboratory Analysis - Second Edition; Approved Standard 1992, NCCLS Document H11-A2.

Procedures for the Collection of Diagnostic Blood Specimens by Skin Puncture - Third Edition; Approved Standard 1991, NCCLS Document H4-A3.

Procedures for the Collection of Diagnostic Blood Specimens by Venepuncture - Third Edition; Approved Standard 1992, NCCLS Document N3-A3.

Procedures for the Handling and Processing of Blood Specimens; Approved Guideline 1990, NCCLS Document H18-A.

Routine Urinalysis and Collection, Transportation, and Preservation of Urine Specimens; Approved Guideline 1995, NCCLS Document GP160A.

Safety in Health Service Laboratories: The labelling, transport and reception of samples 1986; Health Services Advisory Committee, HSE Books, Sudbury, UK.

Selecting and Evaluating a Referral Laboratory; Tentative Guideline 1991, NCCLS Document GP9-T.

Sweat Testing: Sample Collection and Quantitative Analysis; Approved Guideline 1994, NCCLS Document C34-A.

Sykes S. and Goodall I, Interference in Clinical Biochemistry: 'Exploring the Brain-to-Brain Loop'. Clin Biochem Revs 1990: **11**; 144-149.

Wilkinson M, Carrier requirements for Laboratory Samples. Drug Information Journal 1994; **28**;381-384.

COMPUTER

A guide to Managing the Configuration of Computer Systems (Hardware, Software and Firmware) used in NAMAS Accredited Laboratories 1993, NIS 37, Edition 1, NAMAS.

Anderson R, Clinical System Security: Interim Guidelines, BMJ 1996; **312**:109-111.

Laboratory Assessment Checklist, Computer Services Section 1991, Commonwealth Department of Health (Australia), National Pathology Accreditation Council.

Laboratory Instruments and Data Management Systems: Design of Software User Interfaces and End-User Software Systems Validation, Operation and Monitoring; Approved Guideline 1995, NCCLS Document GP19-A.

Recommended Standards for Hospital Laboratory Computer Systems 1986, Liaison Committee on Hospital Laboratory Computing, Dublin, The Academy of Med Lab Sci, Assoc. of Clin. Bioch, Ireland, Pathology Faculty, Roy. Coll. of Physicians in Ireland.

Storage, Transportation and Maintenance of Magnetic Media 1990, NIS 40, NAMAS. (UK).

The application of the principles of GLP to computerised systems. Environmental Monograph No 116, 1995 OECD Paris.

Use of Word Processing Systems in NAMAS Accredited Laboratories 1991, NIS 41, Edition 1, NAMAS (UK).

Chapter 10

Operating process activities — the analytical phase

INTRODUCTION

In this chapter the focus is on the analytical phase of operating process activities and on the management and use of consumables, reagents, calibration and quality control material. There is also a section on near patient testing, which is an operating process activity outside the laboratory but which in St Elsewhere's Hospital Trust is under the overall control of the pathology laboratory.

In Figure 9.1 the stages in the 'Brain-to-Brain Loop' were identified with the preanalytical, analytical and postanalytical phases of operating process activities and in the right hand column the phases were divided into clearly defined steps. In the previous chapter it was pointed out that stage 7 of the 'Brain-to-Brain Loop' occurs in both the preanalytical and analytical phases. This is so that preparation in the sense of 'data acquisition from specimens' can be distinguished from preparation as 'specimen preparation'.

ANALYTICAL — SPECIMEN PREPARATION

In each department of pathology there will be differences in the procedures for the preparation of specimens. In histopathology and cytopathology it is difficult to know whether specimen preparation should be regarded as being separate from the analysis. Certainly the guidelines used in histopathology for 'cut up' or 'gross examination' of specimens prior to embedding are a key part of the analytical process and contribute to the final report in terms of the macroscopic appearance. Similarly, the preparation of blood films in haematology and their subsequent fixation and staining is also a major part of the analytical process.

In haematology and biochemistry a specimen/sample is collected for a specific purpose and it is easy to relate that sample to the original request form by giving the sample and the request form a unique accession number. The problems arise when aliquots of the original sample have to be taken because the analyses required are done on two different analysers. One aliquot might go on an analyser which reads a bar coded label and another onto an analyser where its identity is preserved by relating its order on a work sheet to its position on the carousel. However it is relatively unusual in haematology and biochemistry for extra investigations to be required which were not prescribed in the original request. An example would be if the preliminary analysis of a blood sample on the main haematology analyser revealed some abnormal concentration of a particular group of white cells which it would be necessary to refer for microscopic evaluation, or in biochemistry when an initial measurement of alkaline phosphatase triggered a requirement for isoenzyme analysis.

Developments in instrumentation mean that the primary collection container (often an evacuated tube in which the blood sample is collected) can, after centrifugation to separate the serum from the cellular components, be put directly onto the analytical instrument. Whenever this procedure is possible it should be encouraged, as it reduces the opportunity for errors that occur when aliquots of the original sample have to be put into secondary containers prior to analysis. Such systems will often require the attachment of a bar code label to the primary collection container. This is then 'read' by the analytical instrument, which via a bi-directional interface seeks information from the laboratory computer as to which tests to perform (see Figure 9.19).

However, in microbiology and histopathology it is not always clear until after the initial investigation which subsequent investigations will be required, when a urine is submitted for culture or a specimen is sent for histological examination. It is very important to develop a system in which any subsequent investigations can be related to the original specimen presented for examination. For example, a urine might be cultured and three distinct colonies of micro-organism require further investigation for identification and also for sensitivity testing. A similar situation occurs in histopathology when one or more biopsy specimens are submitted for investigation. Figure 10.1 shows a typical scenario, Step 1: a request form is received with two biopsy specimens, Step 2: two blocks of tissue are prepared from specimen 1 and placed in separate cassettes for embedding, Step 3: paraffin block A is sectioned at two levels to produce sections which are mounted on two slides. It is important to distinguish 'blocks of tissue' from 'paraffin blocks' because Specimen 2 might produce more than one block of tissue, all mounted in one paraffin block.

ANALYTICAL PHASE — ANALYSIS

The laboratory procedures for the analytical phase will cover a wide range of different functions, from the identification of mycobacterium in cerebral spinal fluid to the measurement of serum thyroid stimulating hormone. In this section general issues relating to the structure of such procedures will be discussed, based upon the recommendations of the NCCLS, the International Federation of Clinical Chemistry (IFCC) and NCAAP. Key references are given in Further Reading.

The criteria established in Chapter 4 for the preparation and control of documents should be followed and the first two pages of each procedure will follow the format illustrated in Figures 4.10 and 4.11. The structure of the contents page is illustrated in Figure 10.2 and is

STEP	ACTIVITY	LABELLING	NUMBERING
STEP 1	Request form received with two biopsy specimens	Accession number label for patient request card	96-03066
	Specimen 1	The patient's name etc. should be on the	96-03066-1
	Specimen 2	specimen container label upon receipt, but have accession number labels attached.	96-03066-2
STEP 2	Two blocks of tissue prepared from Specimen 1 and placed in separate cassettes for embedding as:-		
	Paraffin Block A	Paraffin block label	96-03066-1-A
	Paraffin Block B	Paraffin block label	96-03066-1-B
STEP 3	Sections cut from level 1 in Paraffin Block A and mounted on **Slide**	Slide number	96-03066-1-A-1 plus patient's name
	Sections cut from level 2 in Paraffin Block A and mounted on **Slide**	Slide number	96-03066-1-A-2 plus patient's name

Index to number code e.g.   96-03066-2-A-1

96 = year   **03066** = serial accession number   **2** = specimen number
  A = embedding block letter   **1** = level position in block

Figure 10.1   Continuity of identification in histopathology

a development of Figure 4.12. This content is intended to include all the issues that arise in a quantitative method and will need adjusting for qualitative and semi-quantitative methods.

1.0	Purpose and Scope	
2.0	Responsibility	
3.0	References	
4.0	Definitions	
5.0	Documentation	
6.0	Action and methods	

6.1 Principles of the analytical method

6.2 Specimen requirements

6.3 Data acquisition

6.4 Reagents, standards or calibrators, quality control materials- Special supplies and equipment

6.5 Calibration (if appropriate)

6.6 Stepwise description of the procedure (including calculations)

6.7 Quality control and quality assessment

6.8 Limitations of the method

6.9 Reporting of results and clinical interpretation

6.10 Procedure notes and other pertinent information

Figure 10.2   Main headings for the content of an analytical procedure

TITLE

It is important that the title of the procedure gives a clear indication of its purpose, and it is helpful if the title gives some indication of the type of specimen, the method, and instrumentation used. An example might be Procedure for the identification of mycobacteria in cerebral spinal fluid (CSF), Procedure for the measurement of thyroid stimulating hormone (TSH), or Procedure for the measurement of sodium and potassium in serum by direct ion-selective electrode analysis.

PURPOSE AND SCOPE

This section gives the opportunity to describe briefly the clinical context in which the investigation is required, and to whom it should be applied. Two examples are shown, one for the measurement of serum TSH on the BHM analyser and the other for the Gram stain procedure (Figure 10.3).

This procedure for the measurement of TSH could apply to all serum samples received in the laboratory. If there was also a procedure for the measurement of thyroid stimulating hormone on eluates of filter paper blood spots, applicable only to neonatal screening, that

This procedure describes the measurement of Thyroid Stimulating Hormone (TSH) which is a glycoprotein consisting of 2 alpha and 2 beta sub-units. The alpha sub-units are identical to the alpha units of FSH, LH and HCG while the beta sub-units differ. TSH is synthesised in the pituitary and its release is stimulated by thyrotrophin releasing hormone (TRH) secreted from the hypothalamus. TSH synthesis is subject to negative feedback control by the thyroid hormones. TSH stimulates the synthesis and release of T4 and T3 from the thyroid gland. Because of this key role it is used in conjunction with T4 and T3 measurement in the assessment of the integrity of the hypothalamic/pituitary/thyroid axis.

Anon (1996)

The Gram stain ranks among the most important stains for bacteria. It was devised by Christian Gram in 1844, and it allows the microbiologist to broadly distinguish between various bacteria that may exhibit a similar morphology. On microscopic examination of a Gram-stained smear, the differential features of the method will become apparent. Many bacteria will have retained the crystal violet-iodine combination and stain purple (gram-positive) while others will have stained red by the counterstain (gram-negative). Thus, in using this procedure not only are the form, size, and other structural details made visible, but the micro-organisms present can be grouped artificially into gram-positive and gram-negative types by their reactions. This is an important diagnostic tool in subsequent identification procedures.

from Clinical Laboratory Technical Procedure Manuals NCCLS GP2-A2 (1992)

Figure 10.3 Purpose and scope of a laboratory procedure

procedure would indicate that the method was restricted to paediatric samples. Similarly methods which are appropriate for measurement of serum bilirubin in adults may not be applicable to paediatric samples, and the purpose and scope section would need to make that clear.

RESPONSIBILITY
This section should refer to who has the responsibility for implementation of this procedure. In some situations it may be necessary to indicate the required qualifications or position of the individuals. It may be that some of the 'actions and methods' can be performed by a laboratory aide and this should also be made clear.

REFERENCES/DEFINITIONS
The References section should give references to significant published papers describing this method, but if the method has been developed in-house then a reference should be given to documentation which describes the design, development and validation of the method. In ISO 9001:1994 this type of work is covered by clause 4.4. This will be referred to further in the section on method development and validation design. It may be helpful to give some definition of abbreviations to be used throughout the procedure, e.g. TSH

for thyroid stimulating hormone, FIA for fluorescent immunoassay, if that is the particular method used.

DOCUMENTATION

Documentation will refer to any forms that can be used in conjunction with this procedure whether hard copy for bench use or a form of entry on the laboratory computer. Under certain quality and accreditation schemes all raw data has to be retained. (See Figure 10.5 giving the documentation and records associated with the performance of a TRH suppression test and measurement of serum TSH).

ACTION AND METHODS

PRINCIPLE OF THE ANALYTICAL METHOD

This section should include information about the scientific and instrumental principles of the method, and it may be helpful to include reaction sequences in this section. The IFCC guidelines for Preparation of Laboratory Precision Manuals for Clinical Chemistry regard it as appropriate to refer in this section to possible interferences and problems which arise from the inappropriate collection, preservation, and stabilisation of specimens. There is no fixed rule about these matters providing the issues are covered and are accessible. Recommendations regarding the correct specimen containers and interferences appear in the users handbook (Figure 9.3 Section 5) against the entry of a particular test or procedure. In this presentation, interferences would be dealt with in the section on limitations, and problems arising from inappropriate specimen collection under the section on specimen requirements.

SPECIMEN REQUIREMENTS

The NCCLS Clinical Laboratory Technical Procedure Manuals document characterises specimen requirements in three parts, conditions for patient preparation, type of specimen, and handling conditions. The section on conditions for patient preparation refers to instructions on fasting and special diets, and any written instructions which can be given to the patient. It may be that the collection procedure is complicated and associated with a dynamic function test, and reference should be made to an appropriate clinical procedure. Peak and trough measurements of certain antibiotics are required to confirm therapeutic efficacy and this could be included as part of the description of patient preparation, or referenced to another information source. Succinct information is required as to the type of specimen required for the method, the amount required, and acceptable collection containers. If there is a question concerning the stability of the specimen, requirements for storage should be clearly stated. Criteria for unacceptable specimens must be defined, together with the action to be taken by the laboratory. Perhaps the most irritating thing for doctors is to send a sample to the laboratory and have a report sent out some days later saying that the specimen was unsuitable. It is important that immediate action should be taken to inform the doctor if an unsuitable specimen is received by the laboratory. Details may be required regarding handling, transport, and storage conditions, for example serum needing to be separated from the blood within one hour of collection, or a blood sample for blood culture being refrigerated until inoculation. The NCCLS has produced a number of guidelines concerning collection of samples (see Chapter 9, Further Reading).

DATA ACQUISITION

If the laboratory has a computer system, mention should be made of the programme for entering test request data and the mnemonics to be used for particular tests or groups of test. If the specimen has some identifiable problems such as haemolysis, this data can be entered at this stage. If the acquisition and assignment of identity is complex (see Figure 10.1 for histopathology) details of how to proceed at each stage should be given.

REAGENTS, STANDARDS OR CALIBRATORS, QUALITY CONTROL MATERIAL — SPECIAL SUPPLIES AND EQUIPMENT

The NCCLS guideline mentions under the section on reagents or media, special supplies or equipment that the following information should be given: the name, chemical formula, or special ingredients where it is possible, and the acceptable grade. It is also important to refer very clearly to any health or safety information that might be associated with any reagent, supplies, equipment or materials used in the procedure, and giving a class of hazard, e.g. toxic, corrosive, represents a fire hazard, or might be carcinogenic. If referring to prepared reagents or media, or reagent kits, then the supplier should be clearly stated.

With regard to preparation of media or reagents, instructions should be given for the preparation and acceptance criteria prior to use. Parameters used to describe acceptable performance should be stated. Labelling should include a description of the material, lot number, date of preparation and expiry date, and any special storage instructions, e.g. if it should be kept in an explosion-proof refrigerator. Directions for preparing standards should be clearly delineated. The material from which the standards are prepared should include the name and chemical formula, acceptable grade, and the name of the supplying company. As with other reagents there should be information including the type of container, temperature for storage, stability and labelling.

CALIBRATION (IF APPROPRIATE)

With regard to calibration, there should be a detailed stepwise instruction as to how to prepare working standards, preferably enhanced by tabulation. The frequency with which calibration procedures should be performed should be mentioned, and if the method shows calibration results in photometric readings, limits of acceptance should be given. If, in order to calculate the results, a graph is to be prepared then it is important to give an example of the calibration graph.

STEPWISE DESCRIPTION OF THE PROCEDURE

The stepwise description of the method will vary considerably according to whether it is a quantitative testing procedure or a qualitative procedure. In preparation of the stepwise procedure it is useful to prepare a draft and check whether the sequence of steps is as originally drafted. The NCCLS report gives useful examples of both qualitative and quantitative procedures. The instructions should be in a very clear form and kept free of extraneous matter which can much more easily be put under the section on Procedure Notes and other pertinent information. An example for a Gram stain procedure is given in

(1) Cover the heat-fixed smear with the crystal violet solution, allowing the stain to remain for 15 seconds.

(2) Decant crystal violet and rinse slide with iodine until clear.

(3) Flood the slide with the iodine solution for 15 seconds.

(4) Rinse gently with flowing tap water.

(5) Treat with decolorizer solution by flowing the reagent dropwise over the smear while the slide is held at an angle. Stop the decolorization as soon as the dripping from the slide becomes clear.

(6) Remove the excess decolorizer with a gentle flow of water.

(7) Apply the basic fuchsin counterstain for 30 seconds and remove the excess with a gentle flow of tap water.

(8) Drain the slide and blot dry with bibulous paper.

(9) Examine the smear microscopically using the oil immersion objective.

from NCCLS Document GP2-A2 (1992)

Clinical Technical Procedure Manuals - Second Edition

Figure 10.4 Stepwise actions for a Gram stain

Figure 10.4. In this case the instruction for preparation of the smear prior to staining is given in the specimen requirements section.

Some situations can be very complex, for example the BHM analyser (Figure 7.17) is not very advanced and works in batch mode. It will accept samples for measurement of TSH and the same samples can be run again for free thyroxine assay. The ABC laboratory computer produces a worklist which identifies patient samples and quality control samples required for a particular batch, and leaves spaces for the results to be entered. The sample is an aliquot of the original specimen, and the only way in which to identify a specimen on the analyser is to load it in the same order as on the worklist. Such a stepwise procedure would involve information regarding the analyser, computer and reagents/quality control and need careful checking at each step in its preparation.

QUALITY CONTROL/QUALITY ASSESSMENT

A major part of any method is the performance of quality control checks. Quality control is a term that has been misused consistently in the literature over a long period of time, and it is therefore important to define the difference between quality control and quality assessment. Figure 10.5 gives a useful definition of quality control which indicates its role and limitations.

Figure 11.14 in Chapter 11 gives a definition of quality assessment from the same source. Quality control material used in a quantitative assay such as the measurement of TSH, provides an estimate of imprecision at different analyte levels whereas quality control in the case of a Gram stain provides confirmation that it is working. The source of the quality control material must be stated and the batch number and expiry date as appropriate. It is essential that this data is recorded in such a way that it can be associated with the quality control and patient results on a particular day.

Internal quality control...

is the set of procedures undertaken by the staff of a laboratory for continuously assessing laboratory work and the emergent results, in order to decide whether they are reliable enough to be released (either in support of clinical decision making or for epidemiological or research purposes). Thus quality control procedures have an immediate effect on the laboratory's activities and should actually control, as opposed to merely examining the laboratory's output.

WHO External Assessment of Health Laboratories (1981)

Figure 10.5 Definition of internal quality control

The paragraph on quality assessment should indicate which external quality assessment schemes are used to monitor performance of a particular assay. It is desirable that where possible a laboratory belongs to at least two quality assessment schemes for each analyte, and frequency of participation and type of samples should be stated.

LIMITATIONS OF THE METHOD

It is important to introduce in this section any information which could cause interference in the method. This might relate to interference due to lipaemia, haemolysis, high bilirubin content, or effects of drugs whether an in vivo effect on the analyte in question, or an in vitro effect on the assay itself. Details should be given of any foodstuffs or drinks which might cause problems in the assay. It is important to detail any cross-reaction by other compounds or metabolites which occur in both health and disease states.

REPORTING OF RESULTS AND INTERPRETATION

The reporting of quantitative results is straightforward and includes the measurement made, the unit of measurement, and the appropriate reference intervals by sex and age where appropriate. Often there is limited space on a report form, and although certain authorities say that the magnitude of measurement should be included, this may be impractical and best presented in the Users Handbook. Remarks as to likely interferences should be included, although in some instances where the measurement made is known to be severely affected, the comment might be more specific and the result not given. Interpretative comments can be included and form a major part of the report in some disciplines. The procedure should document who or what grade of staff is eligible to report and interpret results.

PROCEDURE NOTES AND OTHER PERTINENT INFORMATION

In this section any pertinent information from any source may be included providing it is completely referenced.

METHOD DEVELOPMENT AND VALIDATION

The majority of methods used in pathology laboratories will have reached a stage where method development within the laboratory is either unnecessary or impractical, e.g. the multilayer dry chemistry systems which are closed and vitiate any possibility of development. However, pathology laboratories should continue to develop and improve upon methodology, as well as introduce new methods. It is necessary under those circumstances for further documentation to be available indicating the development and validation that has taken place.

Requirements in relation to method development (design, etc.) are given in ISO 9001:1994 Clause 4.4 Design, and in EN 45001:1989 5.4.1 Test methods and procedures, where it states 'Where it is necessary to employ test methods and procedures which are non standard, these shall be fully documented.' The NCCLS provides a number of guidelines for method development and validation and these are given in Further Reading.

DOCUMENTATION IN RELATION TO AN ANALYTICAL PROCEDURE

The documentation and records for the situation where serum TSH measurements are made during a thyroid releasing hormone (TRH) suppression test are given in Figure 10.6.

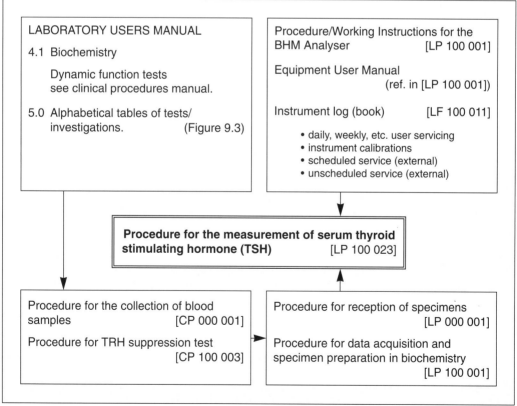

Figure 10.6 Documentation and records for measurement of serum TSH in a TRH suppression test

ORGANISATION OF PROCEDURES FOR OPERATING PROCESS ACTIVITIES

This text uses the term 'Laboratory procedure manual' to describe the organised collection of laboratory procedures which relate to the major part of the procedures required for operating process activities (the exception are procedures involving direct activity with the patient termed clinical procedures and forming the clinical procedures manual). The IFCC reference uses the same term as this text, whereas the NCCLS uses the term 'Laboratory Technical Procedure Manuals' and the NPAAC the term 'Laboratory Manuals' to describe the collections of laboratory procedures. This section develops the concept of an overall structure for documentation which was started in Chapter 4. It shows that laboratory procedures make up the laboratory procedure manual and indicates that the manual, although conceptually one entity, needs to be organised in different volumes or sections for practical reasons.

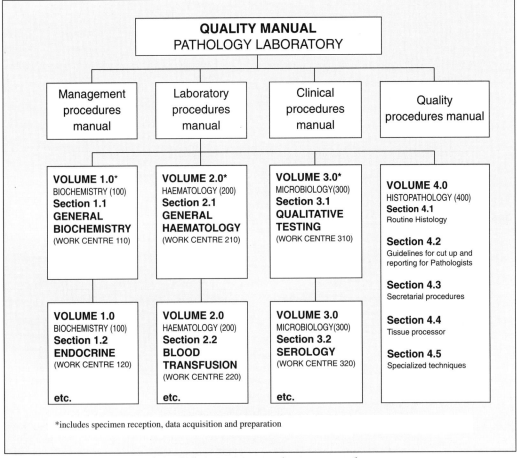

Figure 10.7   Structure of the laboratory procedures manual

The documentation required for the analytical phase of operating process activities and its maintenance is a major undertaking for any laboratory and all quality and accreditation systems require such documentation. In a Pathology laboratory which has chosen to have a unitary structure for its documentation, that is to say, one Quality Manual with supplementary manuals for management, clinical, quality and laboratory procedures (see Figure 4.2); it should be possible to have one management procedure manual for the whole of pathology, but the laboratory procedures manual is likely to have separate volumes for each discipline in pathology unless the laboratory is extremely small.

In some disciplines the particular volume of the laboratory procedure manual can have a number of sections within the one volume as in histopathology, or physically separate sections as shown for biochemistry, haematology and microbiology (see Figure 10.7 for a diagrammatic presentation based on the family tree structure developed in Figure 3.2).

These sections will relate to the way in which the department or discipline is organised, e.g. in biochemistry there may be a section for the work centre 'general biochemistry' and for 'endocrine assays' etc., and microbiology may have separate sections for 'qualitative testing' and 'serology.' In addition to the procedures for the analytical phase of operating process activities, the laboratory procedures manual will also contain any preanalytical and postanalytical laboratory procedures. If they apply to more than one department then copies should be available in the appropriate volumes. It is helpful to design the whole structure of the volumes of the laboratory procedures manual with particular attention to the indexing.

REQUIREMENTS FOR THE ANALYTICAL PHASE OF OPERATING PROCESS ACTIVITIES

The requirements for the analytical phase of operating process activities in the different quality and accreditation schemes are shown in Figure 10.8.

System	Analytical phase of operating process activities
ISO 9001:1994	*(see Figure 9.9 and 9.10 for further information)*
EN 45001:1989	**5 Technical competence** **5.4 Working procedures** *5.4.1 Test methods and procedures* 'The testing laboratory shall have adequate documented instructions on the use and operation of all relevant equipment, on the handling and preparation of test items (where applicable), and on standard testing techniques...' All instructions, standards, manuals and reference data relevant to the work of the testing laboratory shall be maintained up-to-date and be readily available to the personnel. Where it is necessary to employ test methods and procedures which are non-standard, these shall be fully documented.

OECD - GLP	**7. Standard Operating Procedures** **7.1 General** (1) A test facility should have written Standard Operating Procedures approved by management that are intended to ensure the quality and integrity of the data generated in the course of the study. (2) Each separate laboratory unit should have immediately available Standard Operating Procedures relevant to the activities being performed therein. Published text books, articles and manuals may be used as supplements to these Standard Operating Procedures.
CAP - LAP	**Standard IV Quality control** in the interpretation of the standard it says:-'Procedure manuals should follow a standard format and indicate sources, dates of adoption, and evidence of periodic review as described in the National Committee on Clinical Laboratory Standards' (NCCLS) Clinical Laboratory Technical Procedure Manual - Second Edition; Approved Guideline (GP2-A2, 1992)'. 'Methods and instruments shall be validated when introduced and when reintroduced following correction of an "out of control" situation. A complete quality control program must include regular preventive maintenance and appropriate function checks'.
CPA(UK)Ltd	**D Policies and procedures** **D8** There is a written, signed and dated procedure for the performance of each test.

Figure 10.8   Requirements for the analytical phase of operating process activities

MANAGEMENT AND USE OF CONSUMABLES, REAGENTS, CALIBRATION AND QUALITY CONTROL MATERIAL

The proper management of consumables, reagents, calibration and quality control material has an important function in support of their use in operating process activities. A pathology laboratory would normally call the organisation who provided these materials the supplier, but in ISO 9001:1994 the term 'supplier' is equivalent to the pathology laboratory (see Figure 9.9) and the 'subcontractor' is used to denote the supplier of goods or materials. This usage will be adopted in this text and the goods or materials such as the consumables, reagents etc. purchased by the laboratory will be called 'purchased products'. In the text that follows, the terms 'verification' and 'validation' are used in a specific way and in the previous chapter the term validation was used in the context of validation of laboratory reports and the functionality of computers. Figure 10.9 gives the ISO 8402:1994 definitions in relation to quality issues. These definitions are not easy to understand and are best described as, when ordering an item, perhaps a new batch of internal quality control material, certain requirements will have been specified such as expiry date, bottle size, and level of analyte and variance etc. Verification is checking upon receipt to ascertain that you get what was ordered by examining the labelling or package inserts etc. Validation requires, in the case of internal quality control material, using the material to see that the levels specified are within the variance specified, and that it therefore meets the requirements for intended use.

As indicated in the opening sentence of this paragraph there are two separate but interrelated issues concerning consumables, reagents, calibration and quality control material. Firstly the management issues, the way they are procured (ordered, purchased, delivered), verified on receipt and stored prior to use and secondly the operating process activities, how they are issued, validated for use and their use recorded. At all stages in the cycle, records must be kept. On the management side this is important for inventory control and financial management, and on the operational process side it is important for

---

Verification

Confirmation by examination and provision of objective evidence that specified requirements have been fulfilled

Validation

Confirmation by examination and provision of objective evidence that the particular requirements for a specific intended use are fulfilled

ISO 8402:1994
Quality management and quality assurance - Vocabulary

Figure 10.9 Definitions of verification and validation

quality assurance purposes and in order to establish an audit trail which will allow the reconstruction of what consumables, reagents, calibration and quality control material were used when a particular batch of assays were performed. Clause 4.6 of ISO 9001:1994 is entitled 'Purchasing' and is shown in Figure 3.5 as a support activity. Purchasing in the context of the standard includes evaluation of subcontractors, records of purchasing data and the verification of the purchased product. The NCCLS have produced an approved guideline entitled 'Inventory Control Systems for Laboratory Supplies' GP-6 (1994) which describes four phases of inventory control, planning, system development, procurement, and management.

Drawing upon the ISO and NCCLS sources, Figure 10.10 attempts to bring these two interrelated areas together. It follows that a procedure for the management of purchased products is required, a large part of which concerns an inventory system. It is also necessary to either have a laboratory procedure for the validation and use of materials in operating process activities, or to have clear instructions in the appropriate parts of any laboratory procedure which uses such material. For example, such information might be found in sections 6.4, 6.5 and 6.7 of Figure 10.2.

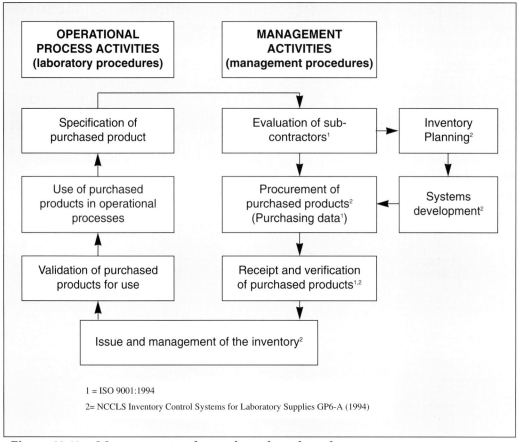

Figure 10.10   Management and use of purchased products

EVALUATION OF SUBCONTRACTOR

The quality system ISO 9001:1994 requires that there should be an evaluation of subcontractors. The pathology laboratory and/or the parent body should be involved in evaluating and selecting subcontractors on their ability to meet the clearly defined requirements of the product(s) being purchased. It is important to record the basis on which subcontractors are selected, which might be one of the following: proof that the subcontractor was registered in an appropriate quality assurance system, the fact that the subcontractor was the sole supplier of a particular product or service, and finally that the subcontractor had a proven record of reliability without being in a quality assurance system. It is required that the extent of control exercised by the laboratory over the subcontractor should be defined and also that records should be kept of the approved subcontractors.

INVENTORY PLANNING AND SYSTEM DEVELOPMENT

The NCCLS document gives a valuable description of how to establish an inventory for laboratory supplies and stipulates a basic analysis in terms of which department in pathology will require which purchased products. It not only requires details for each item but also a view of approximate usage per month, whether the priority of the item is high, medium or low, delivery time, where it will be stored, and under what conditions. A basic structure of an inventory will include information about the subcontractor, the individual items, and ideally specific information on a particular batch in a delivery, the batch number and expiry date, and financial information (Figure 10.11).

PROCUREMENT OF SUPPLIES/RECEIPT AND VERIFICATION

The management procedure should lay down the mechanism for procurement, delivery and receipt, verification and storage of materials. The purchasing documents need to contain data which clearly describes the product ordered and include where applicable the type, class, grade or other precise identification of the material (Figure 10.11). As described earlier

---

Subcontractor (Supplier, vendor)
- Name
- Address
- Telephone number
- Facsimile number

Financial information
- Unit cost
- Discount agreement
- Special tax
- Delivery charges

Individual items
- Description of item
- Part number, catalogue number
- Unit of count
- Usage per month
- Priority
- Procurement lead time
- Storage place and conditions
- Location of use (department, work centre test site)

Specific batch information
- Batch code number
- expiry date
- Number of units
- Date issued

Figure 10.11 Description of purchased products

ISO 9001:1994 requires verification of the purchased product and allows that this can take place on receipt in the laboratory, at the subcontractors premises, or by the customer. The latter two options would be uncommon in the case of a laboratory.

ISSUE AND MANAGEMENT OF THE INVENTORY

This is a further part of an effective stock control and financial management procedure, and the responsibilities for issuing need to be clearly defined. The responsibility for purchasing, delivery, receipt, and issue of materials will be to some extent negotiated with the parent organisation, as some items such as stationery might be purchased by the parent body and supplies obtained by internal requisition. To maintain control of financial expenditure the parent body might be regarded as a subcontractor on the inventory system.

VALIDATION, USE AND SPECIFICATION OF REQUIREMENT OF PURCHASED PRODUCTS

On the operational process activity side (Figure 10.10), a requirement for validation of materials prior to use is a familiar procedure in relation to introducing new reagents, media, quality control items etc. into an operating process and a distinction between validation and verification was drawn earlier. For example, it would be important to check against certain criteria for the receipt of commercially prepared microbiology culture media, and the NCCLS have produced guidelines for quality assurance of commercially prepared microbiological media prior to use (see Further Reading).

Related to this is the effect of information gained in the operational use of purchased products upon the continuing update of the specification for materials to be purchased. If the subcontractor, for example, was asked to provide all quality control material from one single batch to fulfil a requirement for one year of laboratory operation, then a failure to meet this specification would mean either reconsideration of specification or renegotiation with the subcontractor.

REQUIREMENTS FOR CONSUMABLES, REAGENTS, CALIBRATION AND QUALITY CONTROL MATERIAL

The requirements for consumables, reagents, calibration and quality control material in the different quality and accreditation schemes are shown in Figure 10.12

System	Consumables, reagents, calibration and quality control material

ISO 9001:1994	**4. Quality system requirements**
	    4.6 Purchasing
	    4.6.1 *General*
	    The supplier shall establish and maintain documented procedures to ensure that the purchased product conforms to specified requirements.
	    (the paragraph headings below give an indication of the requirements of this part of the standard)
	    4.6.2 *Evaluation of subcontractors*
	    4.6.3 *Purchasing data*
	    4.6.4 *Verification of purchased product*

EN 45001:1989	*(No specific requirement)*

OECD - GLP	**4. Apparatus, material and reagents** **4.2 Material** (1) Apparatus and materials used in studies should not interfere with the test systems. **4.3 Reagents** (1) Reagents should be labelled, as appropriate, to indicate source, identity, concentration, and stability information and should include the preparation date, earliest expiration date, specific storage instructions.
CAP - LAP	**Standard IV Quality control** In the interpretation of the standard it says:- Reagents should be labelled, as appropriate, to indicate source, identity, concentration, and stability information and should include the preparation date, earliest expiration date, specific storage instructions.
CPA(UK)Ltd	**D Policies and procedures** **D7** There is a record of all reagents, calibration and quality material. Guidelines: 1. Part of the process of assessment may involve an audit trail. 2. Procedures should give reagent formulations, methods of preparation, and stability or source of purchase. 3. Batch numbers and source of all reagents, calibrants and QC material, should be recorded with details so that this information can be related to those materials used for an individual assay. 4. The purchasing and stock-keeping arrangements ensure that all materials are in-date when used. 5. There should be suitable arrangements for safe disposal of all material.

Figure 10.12 Requirements for consumables, reagents, calibration and quality control material

NEAR-PATIENT TESTING

Near patient or point of care testing has been documented at least since Thomas Willis (1621-1675) wrote of tasting urine to test for glycosuria. Developments in technology, particularly of the so-called dry chemistry over the past fifteen years, have created many opportunities for pathology tests to be performed outside the conventional laboratory. Within a hospital the situations range from urine stick tests in a side room of a ward or blood glucose and glycated haemoglobin measurements in a Diabetic Clinic, to Intensive Care Units with blood gas and electrolyte analysers. In many countries, primary care physicians (general practitioners) will perform urine stick testing and blood glucose measurements; but in the USA in Physician's Office Laboratories (POL's), a wider range of pathology is encompassed.

In the USA under CLIA'88, tests are now divided into waived tests, moderate-complexity and high-complexity tests. A certificate of waiver allows a facility to perform without accreditation a limited range of simple tests, which include certain ovulatory tests or urinary pregnancy tests, faecal occult blood, and blood glucose by monitoring devices that have been cleared by the Federal Drug Administration specifically for home use. The Commission on Office Laboratory Accreditation (COLA) has deemed status under CLIA'88 to accredit POL's and over the past five years has accredited some 7,000 laboratories ranging in size from solo practitioner's offices to large group practices. The accreditation process includes a self assessment against 299 specific questions and the organisation additionally produces excellent educational material in the form of LabGuide's (see Appendix 1 for addresses). The NCCLS publish 'The Physician's Office Laboratory Guidelines' and 'Procedure Manual' (see Further Reading) which contains material which is not only useful to POL's but is worthy of study by directors of conventional laboratories. In particular the material on venepuncture and on collection of other biological specimens would be invaluable in the preparation of procedures.

The Guidelines on the control of near-patient testing and procedures performed on patients by non-pathology staff, produced in the UK by the Joint Working Party on Quality Assurance, require that laboratory staff should be involved in the management of all such facilities in a hospital. The King's Fund Organisational Audit in Primary Health Care (UK) have standards which require liaison with the local accredited laboratory. Near patient testing facilities have often developed because the laboratory service has been poor, particularly in turnaround times. However, in view of the difficulties of maintaining effective control over a situation where blood glucose monitors are in every ward, clinic and special care unit in a hospital and used by doctors and nurses, the first question should be 'Do we need near-patient testing?' The answer will be yes in situations such as intensive care units, but in hospitals with the laboratory manned twenty-four hours a day, pneumatic tube transport to the laboratory, and test result terminals on every ward, the question should be revisited at defined intervals. Further Reading gives a reference to a paper on 'Near-Patient Testing - Management Issues' and the Association of Clinical Biochemists (UK) have produced a pamphlet entitled 'Guidelines for the Implementation of Near-Patient Testing'.

ORGANISATION AND MANAGEMENT

A recent survey of laboratory facilities in one hundred and twenty-five intensive care units showed that 49% did not consult their pathology laboratory regarding choice of equipment or methodology, 30% did no quality control, 46% of Intensive Care Units had no idea how much their laboratory facilities cost to run and 11% carried out more than 100 tests per day. The authors of the report proposed guidelines based upon the CPA(UK)Ltd Standards.

The organisation and management of near-patient testing in a hospital requires the involvement of a number of different professional groups, and the first step is to form a working group or near-patient testing committee. This should normally be chaired by a senior member of the pathology laboratory, and its membership should be drawn from intensive care staff, diabetic nurses, nurse educators, pharmacists, biochemists and, if haematology testing is done, a representative from that department. The main problem in the management of near-patient testing is the very wide spread and diffuse nature of the operation. It is, therefore, important that individual responsibilities be clearly defined, and the working group must meet regularly to review the results of any quality assurance activities.

EQUIPMENT, REAGENTS AND CONSUMABLES

In each section of the procedure for the management of near-patient testing (Figure 10.14) the first subsection requires a definition of responsibilities in relation to the topic of that subsection. An inventory should be kept of all the equipment used for near-patient testing throughout the hospital, and it would be appropriate to make this a subset of the laboratory equipment inventory. Unique identification, particularly of blood glucose meters, needs to be recorded. The arrangements for equipment maintenance should follow the lines of the main laboratory. If equipment in an ICU, such as blood gas and electrolyte analysers, is held in common with the laboratory, it is good practice to have equipment provided by the same manufacturer as this simplifies arrangements for equipment maintenance and enables trained laboratory staff to be available to assist in situations outside the laboratory.

A small but important issue for maintenance of glucose meters, is to know where to get spare batteries. As the unit cost of glucose meters themselves is not prohibitive, the laboratory should have spare meters available so that a malfunctioning meter can be replaced immediately. The staff in the laboratory outside the normal working hours should know the procedure for replacing a blood glucose meter or providing new batteries.

The purchase and issue of reagents and consumables is often complicated by the fact that the pharmacy is responsible for the purchase and issue of urine testing strips, and quite often for blood glucose strips. If this is so, a representative of the pharmacy staff should be a member of the working group, particularly as they are frequently on the wards and, if given the responsibility for purchasing can assist in ensuring that in date and uniform products are used.

STAFF TRAINING

Organisation and content of staff training should be defined by the working group, but the staff actually doing the training can be drawn from a number of different sources. In the case of blood glucose testing, manufacturers often provide good quality training programmes as part of an overall package which also includes quality control and assessment programmes. Diabetic nurses are often required to teach patients how to use a variety of glucose monitors for self-testing, and have a wide range of practical experience which represents an important resource when preparing a training programme.

The content of the training programme should emphasise the importance of quality assurance, and of keeping proper records of patients results and the results of internal quality control and external quality assessment. The form used in St Elsewhere's Hospital for blood glucose results on patients and quality control material is shown in Figure 10.13. Records should be made of the date and time when the sample was collected and analysed. These records should be stored in a designated location in case there is need to check back on a particular result. The injunction at the bottom requires that the form is returned to the laboratory upon completion as part of the quality assurance programme. In addition to entering patients results onto the work sheet they should also be recorded in the patients notes/record with an indication that the result was obtained using a glucose meter.

The attention of staff should be drawn to the health and safety aspects involved in near-patient testing. When a member of staff is trained they should be given an authorised user number and their details entered on a register of authorised users. Through quality assessment schemes (see below) it is possible to monitor an authorised user's performance and assess any need for further training.

PROCEDURES, FORMS AND RECORDS
The working party should be responsible for the preparation of procedures and forms and agree on their suitability before issue. In the near-patient testing situation, the procedure for blood glucose measurements will most likely refer to simple working instructions and manufacturers are often able to produce suitable material on durable laminated card. The NCCLS have produced an approved guideline 'Ancillary (Bedside) Blood glucose Testing in Acute and Chronic Care Facilities'; and a proposed guideline, 'Point-of-Care IVD Testing' which merit careful study.

The importance of recording the patient results on a specially designed form, and in the patient record has been mentioned above with respect to glucose results. The record should contain at a minimum, the name of the patient, the date and time of analysis, the results obtained, the batch number of reagents used and the serial number of the meter. The form shown in Figure 10.13 is designed to facilitate compliance with these requirements.

QUALITY CONTROL AND ASSESSMENT
The organisation of all quality assurance activities is best done in conjunction with the main laboratory. A procedure for a particular test or investigation must give advice on how frequently quality control samples should be used and include guidance on how to determine that the results are satisfactory. In many near-patient situations it is difficult to get suitable material for conventional quality assessment and alternative approaches are important. In the case of blood glucose, with permission from a few selected patients, it is possible to take an extra blood sample into a sodium fluoride bottle at the same time as measuring the blood glucose using a meter. This sample is then sent to the laboratory together with a specially designed request form on which the staff measuring the blood glucose outside the laboratory record their result. Once the relationship between the two

St Elsewhere's Hospital Trust	LF NPT 011
	Edition 1
WORKING PARTY ON NEAR PATIENT TESTING	Page 1/1

BLOOD GLUCOSE FORM

LOCATION	

BLOOD GLUCOSE METER Serial Number	REAGENT BATCH Code Number

QUALITY CONTROL LEVEL 1	QUALITY CONTROL LEVEL 2
Batch Code number	Batch Code number
Acceptable range mmol/L	Acceptable range mmol/L

DATE	TIME	PATIENTS' NAME/HOSPITAL No. or QUALITY CONTROL 1 or 2	RESULTS (mmol/L)	AUTHORISED USER	COMMENTS

PLEASE RETURN TO THE LABORATORY WHEN FORM IS COMPLETED

LABORATORY FORM

Figure 10.13   Near patient testing -blood glucose form

methods of measurement is understood by the laboratory then comparisons between the meter reading and the laboratory assay can be made and the information fed back to the near-patient testing location at regular intervals. With older glucose meters, the meter reading could also be checked by comparing this result with the visual reading of the colour on the test strip against a graduated scale of colours. In the case of measurements of blood gases and electrolytes in the ICU, results should be regularly checked against measurements obtained in the laboratory on an aliquot of the same specimen.

QUALITY AUDIT

In addition to the quality assurance activities already mentioned, a quality audit of all near-patient testing sites in the hospital should be undertaken at least once a year. This may be a time-consuming activity, but nevertheless it is important as it will draw the attention of staff to the fact that the laboratory is monitoring how things are performed. It is helpful if the quality audit designates certain items to be checked, for example in the case of blood glucose to inspect the general area in which testing is done to see that there is good housekeeping and no blood contamination on surfaces or apparatus, or used materials left lying around. The meter can be checked and any quality records examined. The availability of instructions can be checked and staff asked a few general questions designed to indicate their current knowledge.

INTERPRETATION OF RESULTS

Near-patient testing is different from measurements made by the laboratory in that the results are available when the patient is still present. Once reliable results have been produced it is necessary to interpret them so they can be used for patient care. If the results are interpreted by someone other than the patient's doctor, then guidelines need to be written defining what interpretation and advice is to be given. If the results obtained by near-patient testing indicate the need for a significant change in treatment, particularly in the case of blood glucose, the laboratory should be asked to do a confirmatory test. There needs to be a clear arrangement on the availability of expert help in interpretation.

HEALTH AND SAFETY

As mentioned previously, it is important that staff training involves a proper understanding of good housekeeping and health and safety, and this should be undertaken in accordance with properly laid-down guidelines.

PROCEDURE FOR THE MANAGEMENT OF NEAR-PATIENT TESTING.

The contents page of a procedure for the management of near patient testing is given in Figure 10.14.

Content of procedure

1.0   Purpose and Scope

2.0   Responsibility

3.0   References

4.0   Definitions

5.0   Documentation

6.0   Action and methods

6.1 Organisation and management

    6.1.1 Working Group on Near Patient Testing
    6.1.2 Membership
    6.1.3 Frequency of meetings

6.2 Equipment, reagents and consumables

    6.2.1 Responsibilities
    6.2.2 Equipment inventory
    6.2.3 Equipment maintenance
    6.2.4 Purchase and issue of reagents and consumables

6.3 Staff training

    6.3.1 Responsibilities
    6.3.2 Training programme
    6.3.3 Register of authorised users

6.4 Procedures, forms and records

    6.4.1 Responsibilities
    6.4.2 Procedures, working instructions and forms
    6.4.3 Patient records
    6.4.4 Quality records

6.5 Quality Assurance

    6.5.1 Responsibilities
    6.5.2 Quality control
    6.5.3 Quality assessment
    6.5.4 Quality audit

6.6   Interpretation of results

6.7   Health and Safety

Figure 10.14   Content of procedure for management of near patient testing

FURTHER READING

ANALYTICAL PHASE OF OPERATING PROCESS ACTIVITIES

An Introduction to Autopsy Technique, 1994, CAP Document BK280.

Autopsy Performance and Reporting, 1990, CAP Document B205.

Clinical Laboratory Technical Procedure Manuals - Second Edition; Approved Guideline 1992, NCCLS Document GP2-A2.

Evaluation of the Linearity of Quantitative Analytical Methods; Proposed Guideline 1986, NCCLS Document EP6-P.

Farcus D H. Molecular Biology and Pathology: A Guidebook for Quality Control, 1993, AACC Press.

Guidelines for the preparation of laboratory manuals 1986, Commonwealth Department of Health (Australia), National Pathology Accreditation Advisory Council.

Guidelines (1988) for preparation of laboratory procedure manuals for clinical chemistry, J of Automatic Chemistry 1989; **11**:32-35.

Internal Quality Control Testing: Principles and Definitions; Approved Guideline 1991, NCCLS Document C24-A.

Inventory Control Systems for Laboratory Supplies; Approved Guideline 1994, NCCLS Document P6-A.

Laboratory Histopathology: A Complete Reference, ed Woods A E, and Ellis R C., 1994, Churchill Livingstone.

Method Comparison and Bias Estimation Using Patient Samples; Approved Guideline 1995, NCCLS Document EP9-A.

Microbiology Self-Instruction Modules,1994
    Module 1: Basic Microbiology Techniques, CAP Document B601.
    Module 2: Throat Culture, CAP Document B602.
    Module 3: Urine Culture, CAP Document B603.
    Module 4: Genital Culture, CAP Document B604.
    Module 5: Skin/Wound Culture, CAP Document B605.

Papanicolaou Technique; Approved Guideline 1994, NCCLS Document GP15-A.

Performance Goals for the Internal Quality Control of Multichannel Hematology Analyzers; Proposed Standard 1989, NCCLS Document H26-P.

Practice Guidelines for Autopsy Pathology: Autopsy Performance. Archives of Pathology and Laboratory Medicine, 1995; CAP Document B281.

Practice Parameter for the Use of Fresh-Frozen Plasma, Cryoprecipitate, and Platelets. Journal of the American Medical Association, 1994, CAP Document B201.

Precision Performance of Clinical Chemistry Devices - Second Edition; Tentative Guideline 1992, NCCLS Document EP5-T2.

Preliminary Evaluation of Quantitative Clinical Laboratory Methods - Second Edition; Tentative Guideline 1993, NCCLS Document EP10-T2.

Protocol for the Examination of Specimens removed from patients with Colorectal Carcinoma: A basis for checklists. Archives of Pathology and Laboratory Medicine, 1994, CAP Document B265.

Quality Assurance for Commercially Prepared Microbiological Culture Media; Approved Standard 1990, NCCLS Document M22-A.

Young, D S. Effects of Drugs on Clinical Laboratory Tests, Fourth Edition, 1995, AACC Press.

NEAR PATIENT TESTING

Ancillary (Bedside) Blood Glucose Testing in Acute and Chronic Care Facilities; Approved Guideline 1994, NCCLS Document C30-A.

Burnett D. and Freedman D. Near-patient testing: The Management Issues, Health Services Management 1994;10-13.

Clinical Laboratory Handbook for Patient Preparation and Specimen Handling: Supplement for Physician Office Laboratories, 1993, CAP Document B220.

Cox D J A. and Naidoo R. The intensive care laboratory - a report of current UK practice and recommendations for the implementation of required minimum standards, Care of the Critically Ill 1995; **11**:98-103.

England J M, Hyde K, Lewis S M, Mackie I J, and Rowan R M. Guidelines for near patient testing: Haematology, Clin Lab Haem 1995; **7**:301-310.

Hicks JM. Near-patient testing: is it here to stay, J Clin Pathol 1996; **49**:191-193

Labelling of Home-Use In Vitro Testing Products; Approved Guideline 1996, NCCLS Document GP14-A.

Physician Office Laboratory Policy and Procedure Manual, 1993, CAP Document B219.

Point-of-Care IVD Testing; Proposed Guideline 1995, NCCLS Document AST2-P.

Chapter 11

Quality assurance and evaluation

INTRODUCTION

Different definitions of quality assurance are given in Figure 11.1, and quality itself has been discussed previously in Chapter 2.

Quality Assurance

'All the planned and systematic activities implemented within the quality system and demonstrated as needed, to provide adequate confidence that an entity will fulfil requirements for quality'

ISO 8402:1994 Quality management and quality assurance-Vocabulary

---

'...in laboratory medicine is the process of assuring that all pathology services involved in the delivery of patient care have been accomplished in a manner appropriate to maintain excellence in medical care'

Glossary - Standards of Laboratory Accreditation
College of American Pathologists (1988)

'...is the practice that encompasses all procedures and activities directed towards ensuring that a specified product is achieved and maintained. In the clinical laboratory, this includes monitoring all the raw materials, supplies, instruments, procedures, sample collection/transport/storage/processing, record keeping, calibration and maintenance of equipment, quality control, proficiency testing, training of personnel, and all else involved in the production of the data reported'

Nomenclature and Definitions for use in NRSCL and NCCLS Documents
Second edition Proposed Guideline NCCLS document NRSCL8-P2 (1993)

'The managed process whereby the comparison of care against predetermined standards is guaranteed to lead to action to implement changes, and ensuring that these have produced the desired improvement'

Donabedian A (1966)

Figure 11.1   Definitions of quality assurance

The ISO 8042:1994 definition of quality assurance is valuable in drawing attention to the need for a planned and systematic approach. The CAP-LAP definition is important as it emphasises the role of laboratory medicine in maintaining excellence in medical care and reminds us that quality assurance must not only be restricted to the analytical aspects of laboratory medicine. The NCCLS definition details some of the things that should be done and represents the beginning of a quality plan. It is not surprising that Donabedian's definition could be read as a definition of clinical audit as it came from an article entitled 'Evaluating the Quality of Medical Care', but it is important also for its emphasis on the requirement for continuous improvement. Donabedian himself did not particularly like the term quality assurance, regarding it as 'too optimistic a term' and spoke more about evaluation and assessment in his seminal works on quality in health-care. The title of this chapter includes the term evaluation. In common usage to evaluate means 'to judge or assess the worth of...' If quality assurance is to 'inspire confidence in the quality of the product' then evaluation is the part of quality assurance that puts the emphasis onto 'Is what we are doing in pathology of value to the doctor/patient?'.

This chapter aims to bring together the requirements of the different quality and accreditation systems with respect to quality assurance, and establish an approach which might meet the different requirements. There are a number of different ways of looking at quality assurance activities. A simplistic way is to look at the activities carried out within the laboratory by the staff themselves such as internal audits, quality control etc., and at the activities of outside agencies in terms of providing external quality assessment or proficiency testing and accreditation to the laboratory. This simplistic approach, however, leaves a number of questions to be answered, e.g. 'Where does clinical audit fit, and are these approaches focused sufficiently on the doctor/patient needs?'

The complexity of terminology in quality assurance requires further discussion before the different aspects of quality assurance can be developed. The 1994 edition of ISO 8402 'Quality management and quality assurance-Vocabulary' greatly expands on the 1986 edition and divides the terms used into four categories. A selection of the terms in each category is shown in Figure 11.2 with their paragraph numbers. Most likely to cause confusion is the way in which certain terms are classified into 'terms relating to quality systems' and to 'tools and techniques'. It can be seen that quality evaluation and surveillance are regarded as tools or techniques, whereas quality control, which laboratory staff would regard as a tool or technique, is in the section on quality system terms. Quality assessment (proficiency testing) is a term also familiar in the pathology laboratory but is not mentioned. However, the notes attached to 'quality surveillance' state that in English, quality surveillance is sometimes called quality assessment, quality appraisal or quality survey.

---

*The Collins English Dictionary 3rd Edition updated 1994 ISBN 0 00 470678-1

1. General terms

1.1 entity or item	1.10 supplier
1.2 process	1.11 purchaser
1.3 procedure	1.12 contractor
1.5 product	1.13 subcontractor
1.6 service	

2. Terms related to quality

2.1 quality	2.10 non conformity
2.3 requirement for quality	2.17 verification
2.4 requirement for society	2.18 validation
2.8 safety	

3. Terms related to quality systems

3.1 quality policy	3.6 quality system
3.2 quality management	3.8 quality improvement
3.3 quality planning	3.9 management review
3.4 quality control	3.12 quality manual
3.5 quality assurance	3.15 quality record

4. Terms related to tools and techniques

4.1 quality loop or spiral	4.9 quality audit
4.6 quality evaluation	4.15 disposition of a non conformity
4.7 quality surveillance	

Figure 11.2 Terminology in quality assurance (with paragraph numbers)

QUALITY CONTROL, SURVEILLANCE, AUDIT, OR EVALUATION?

The introduction to this chapter dealt with some aspects of the terms used in quality assurance. There are a confusing number of different terms used to describe the different approaches to seeing 'that all is well and that it is of value'. In this text the term quality assurance (defined in several ways in Figure 11.1) is used, as the ISO 8402:1994 definition suggests, to include 'all systematic and planned activities implemented within the quality system'. Further international definitions for the key terms used in this text are given in Figure 11.3.

In the Pathology laboratory the terms 'internal quality control' and 'external quality assessment' (proficiency testing) are perhaps the most familiar, although in the past the term 'external quality control' was frequently used instead of external quality assessment. The World Health Organisation (WHO) definition of internal quality control was given in Figure 10.5 and the WHO definition for external quality assessment is given in Figure 11.14.

Quality control

The operational techniques and activities that are used to fulfil requirements for quality.

Quality surveillance (Quality assessment)

The continuing monitoring and verification of the status of an entity, and analysis of records to ensure specified requirements for quality are fulfilled.

Quality audit

Systematic and independent examination to determine whether quality activities and related results comply with planned arrangements and whether these are implemented effectively and are suitable to achieve objectives.

Quality evaluation

Systematic examination of the extent to which an entity is capable of fulfilling specified requirements.

ISO 8402:1994 Quality management and quality assurance-Vocabulary

Figure 11.3 International definitions of quality terms

The essential difference between quality control and quality surveillance (assessment), audit, and evaluation, is the time frame in which remedial action can be taken. For example, if a batch of assays is performed and the results on quality control samples are outside agreed limits, then the results on patient samples can be withheld and the batch repeated. In other words 'the stable door can be closed before the horse has bolted'. On the other hand, if the results on external quality assessment samples are found to be outside acceptable limits then all that can be done is to instigate a retrospective examination of that particular assay. Many horses may have bolted in the meantime! In this text quality control is used in an operational sense and results in 'immediate feedback control'.

The introduction to ISO 8402:1994 draws attention to the use of the words 'assure' and 'ensure', saying that, to ensure is 'to make sure or certain' and assure 'to give confidence to oneself or others'. It is interesting that the definition for quality surveillance uses the word ensure, because if it is the same as quality assessment then it cannot ensure that results are correct, but only retrospectively give assurance that all was well at the time the tests were done. In this sense only quality control can ensure the quality requirements of the product (test result or report in pathology), as by definition it allows immediate remedial action to be taken at the appropriate stage in operational process activities.

The term quality audit, as defined, acts more to assure or inspire confidence in the quality system and associated activities. An important aspect of quality audit and assessment is the element of independence, in that an independent agency is involved. In the case of quality audit this would be the Quality Assurance Unit (QAU) of the laboratory, and for external quality assessment schemes the agency which organises the particular scheme.

All these activities are carried out with the expectation of comparison against some agreed standard, in the case of internal quality control against 'internally agreed limits'. With quality assessment, in the case of quantitative measurements, comparison is against an overall or method mean and the distribution of results, and in qualitative investigations against the 'correct result'. As the definitions state, quality control is carried out 'to fulfil requirements for quality', quality surveillance (assessment) 'in relation to stated references', quality audit against 'planned arrangements', and quality evaluation to see if the entity 'is capable of fulfilling specified requirements'.

ISO 8402:1994 term	Pathology Laboratory activity
Quality control	• Quality control (particularly internal QC)
Quality surveillance	• Quality assessment (particularly external QA or proficiency testing) • Accreditation or Certification
Quality audit	• Quality audit
Quality evaluation	• Management review • Clinical audit

Figure 11.4 Quality terms interpreted for the pathology laboratory

Figure 11.4 equates ISO 8402:1994 terms with those which might be used in the pathology laboratory. Quality evaluation is identified in two distinct ways, as an evaluation of the quality system itself (management review), and as an evaluation of a product as 'fit for a purpose' (clinical audit). Figure 11.5 takes these different quality assurance activities and indicates which group of staff or organisation is involved in each activity. The open diamonds indicate that the QAU has delegated responsibilities to individual disciplines or departments but maintains an overview. Whether organisations operating accreditation schemes also organise proficiency testing/external quality schemes is variable and in Figure 11.5 this altonate is indicated by an open diamond. This topic is discussed later in the chapter.

Pathology Laboratory activity	GROUP OR AGENCIES DIRECTLY INVOLVED IN THE ACTIVITY				
	QA Unit	Laboratory Staff	Service users	EQA schemes	Accreditation agencies
Quality control (particularly internal QC)	◊	♦			
Quality assessment (particularly external QA or proficiency testing)	◊	♦		♦	◊
Certification or accreditation	♦	♦	♦		♦
Quality audit	♦	♦			
Management review	♦	♦			
Clinical audit	◊	♦	♦		

Figure 11.5 Involvement in quality assurance activities

INTEGRATED APPROACH TO QUALITY ASSURANCE

It is apparent from the requirements of different quality and accreditation schemes for quality assurance activity that, unless an integrated approach can be devised that will suit all certifying and accreditation bodies, any laboratory seeking recognition in more than one scheme will be involved in a lot of repetitious work simply to satisfy different agencies. Figure 11.6 is a schematic of the relationship between the different components of quality assurance in which accepted international terminology is used. It embraces quality audit, quality control, quality assessment and clinical audit, requires a customer focus, the maintenance of existing quality, and improvement where necessary. It attempts to bring together all aspects of quality assurance to fulfil all the requirements of the quality and accreditation schemes, and the remainder of this chapter will aim to demonstrate how this might be achieved.

Further Reading includes a report on the experience of developing a quality assurance programme, acceptable for purposes of ISO 9000, NAMAS (now the United Kingdom Accreditation Service and based on EN 45000), and GLP. It also reiterates the requirements of the different systems. 'It is our understanding that the major difference of the three Quality Standards exists in emphasis on different aspects of the analytical process. With GLP being most concerned with data integrity for those analytical studies associated with regulatory submission: NAMAS being most concerned with the traceability studies of calibration and measurement, and the accuracy and validity of the individual analytical measurements, whereas ISO 9001 places major emphasis on the capabilities of the facility to control the analytical process, such that the customers expectations are clearly understood, agreed, and efficiently and effectively delivered'.

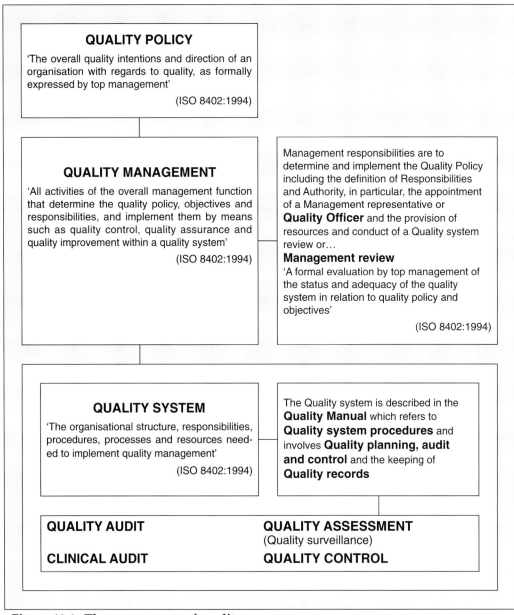

Figure 11.6   The components of quality assurance

MANAGEMENT RESPONSIBILITIES

Most systems require implicitly or explicitly that management appoint a person or persons to be in charge of quality assurance activities, and then define the tasks required to be performed. As discussed in Chapter 5, management is taken to mean the director of the pathology laboratory or the head of a department or discipline. Whatever the nature of the quality system or quality assurance activity there are three key factors for success shown in Figure 11.7. In different systems of accreditation the way in which quality assurance activities are organised and who takes responsibility is broadly the same.

Management must ....

- make a clear commitment to and demonstrate support for the process

- define and document its policy for quality

- appoint a quality officer who can act independently and is responsible to management

---

Figure 11.7   Management's responsibilities in quality assurance

QUALITY POLICY

The importance and role of a quality policy have been discussed in Chapter 5, and examples of policies are given in Figure 5.14 and on page 5/19 of Figure 5.15. It can be seen from Figure 11.6 that the quality policy is the first step in management's commitment to a quality assurance programme.

QUALITY MANAGER

In illustrative opening pages of the Quality Manual, section 2.2 'Organisation and responsibilities within the pathology laboratory' there is a structure showing a QAU with a Quality Manager who is a full member of the Pathology Management Board (Figure 5.15). In a large organisation there may be more than one quality officer and they will work with a quality team. In smaller units it is likely that the quality officer will have other duties to perform and care should be taken to ensure that conflicts do not occur between their role in quality assurance and their role in running a section of the laboratory.

The three international standards (ISO 9001:1994, EN 45001:1989, OECD-GLP) all embrace the concept of a person being designated by management to be in charge of quality assurance activities. In ISO 9001:1994 the individual is described as the 'management representative'. Certain principles emerge from the description of the role (as distinct from their responsibilities) of such a person and these are shown in Figure 11.8.

The Quality Manager ....

- is appointed by management

- reports directly to management

- must be familiar with the work being assured

- should not be involved in the work being assured

Figure 11.8 The role of the quality manager

The general responsibilities of a quality manager, based on the description in ISO 9001:1994, are shown in Figure 11.9. In OECD-GLP, quality assurance personnel have what appear to be special responsibilities in relation to studies study plans and final reports, but with interpretation those can be seen as a specific example of a general case (Figure 9.11).

The responsibilities of the Quality Manager are ....

- to ensure that a quality system is established, implemented and maintained on a day to day basis

- to plan, record, and organise quality audits

- to ensure that deficiencies or noncompliances are corrected in a timely manner

- to report the performance of the quality system to management for review (management review)

- to ensure that any action required as a result of the review is implemented

---

Figure 11.9 The responsibilities of the quality manager

MANAGEMENT REVIEW

In the 1986 version of ISO 8402 the term 'quality system review' was used instead of the term 'management review'. One term indicates who should undertake the review, and the other what it is about. A key part of ISO 9001:1994 is the concept of a management review or quality system review. Remembering that 'supplier' is equivalent to the laboratory, the standard says, 'The supplier's management with executive responsibility shall review the quality system at defined intervals sufficient to ensure its continuing suitability and effectiveness in satisfying the requirements of this International Standard and the supplier's stated quality policy and objectives …Record of such reviews shall be maintained…'. Not surprisingly that definition is very similar to the international definition in ISO 8402:1994,

'A formal evaluation by top management of the status and adequacy of the quality system in relation to quality policy and objectives' and EN 45001:1989 describes an identical process 'The quality system shall be systematically and periodically reviewed by or on behalf of management to ensure the continued effectiveness of the arrangements, and any necessary corrective action initiated. Such reviews shall be recorded together with details of any corrective action taken'. In the CAP-LAP and CPA(UK)Ltd system there is not an explicit requirement to review the quality system itself as distinct from undertaking quality assurance.

At St Elsewhere's this review is conducted on an annual basis by a special meeting of the Management Board of the Pathology Laboratory. This ensures that top management is involved and enables the findings to form the annual report and future objectives of the laboratory (Figure 6.14), which in turn can be used in staff appraisal.

QUALITY SYSTEM AND ORGANISATION

In the previous paragraphs the emphasis has been on the role of management in quality assurance, a top downwards approach. However, no quality activities will succeed unless all staff are involved, and that should be reflected in the organisational arrangements of a quality system. As can be seen in the procedure for the 'Organisation and management of pathology'(Figure 5.11), the Quality Assurance Unit of St Elsewhere's pathology laboratory, like the Health and Safety committee, is a sub committee of the Pathology Management Board, and as such should meet at specified intervals. Its main role will be defined in the procedure governing the conduct of quality assurance in the laboratory.

In addition to the Quality Manager, who might act as chairman of the QAU sub committee, membership should be broadly based to include personnel who have special knowledge of the operational aspects of each department. It is helpful if all staff groups, medical, scientific, technical, administrative and clerical are included. In each department or discipline there should be a quality assurance group which will be responsible for any work delegated by the QAU. These groups should set departmental standards, review results in external quality assessment schemes, co-ordinate and supervise day to day quality control activities, and undertake clinical audit. As with the organisation and management of computing it is important that each discipline has a quality assurance co-ordinator who liaises closely with the quality manager.

QUALITY MANUAL

The requirement for a quality manual in the different quality and accreditation schemes has been given in Figure 4.14, and in Chapter 5 its role, structure and content (Figures 5.12, 5.13 and 5.15) was discussed. As described in Chapter 5, 'it serves to introduce the scope and purpose of the laboratory and its policies, and to create an organisational structure for documentation'.

QUALITY SYSTEM PROCEDURES, PLANNING AND RECORDS

The content of a 'Procedure for the Management of Quality Assurance' is given in Figure 11.22 and it acts as a 'framework' for more specific procedures which might govern, for example, the conduct of 'Clinical Audit in Pathology', or a procedure for the review of 'External Quality Assessment Results in Histopathology'. There is a general requirement in quality and accreditation systems to plan activity and to keep records. Quality assurance is no exception and examples will be given later in this chapter.

QUALITY AUDIT

ORGANISATION AND RESPONSIBILITY

Quality audit concerns the audit of procedures contained in the Quality Manual (and its related volumes). Figure 11.10 indicates the essential requirements for quality audit. The quality manager is responsible for ensuring that audits take place and in a small department will be able to undertake most of the audits concerned with pathology-wide procedures, but in larger departments it will be necessary to nominate suitably trained members of staff to assist the quality manager.

Quality audits are part of the quality system and are.....

- conducted in accordance with a pre-planned programme

- by a nominated person who does not have direct responsibility in the area being audited

- at a specified time

- according to documented procedure and the results are recorded

- reviewed at the Quality Manager/QAU sub-committee, non conformities being identified and a reasonable timescale for remedial action agreed

---

Figure 11.10 Requirements for quality audits

PURPOSE OF AUDITS

The major purpose of quality audits is to establish that the management's objectives as defined in the quality system are being fulfilled, that all staff carry out their assigned duties and responsibilities, and that the procedures detailed in the quality manual are being followed. Inspection of the proposed contents of the management procedures described in this text will indicate that audit activity is an inherent part of these procedures. Relevant examples are given in Figure 5.11, Annual Review of Objectives (organisation and management); Figure 6.16, Joint review (personnel management); Figure 7.19 Assessment and justification of need (equipment management); Figure 8.11 Risk assessment, Monitoring and audit (health and safety).

PLANNING, IMPLEMENTATION AND RECORDS

It is essential to have a schedule for the conduct of quality audits, and the schedule for audit of management procedures in St Elsewhere's Pathology Laboratory is shown in Figure 11.11. At the bottom of the form is the key to progress on the schedule.

In the case of St Elsewhere's there are management, laboratory and clinical procedures and their forms to be audited. The quality audit ascertains whether they are current, they are being followed, and that there is evidence that they are being followed? In addition, any quality procedures specified in the 'framework' procedure for quality assurance must be audited. Records of the audits undertaken must be kept and any non conformities or matters requiring improvement identified. A non conformity is the 'nonfulfilment of a specified requirement'*, and disposition of a non conformity is the 'action taken to deal with a non conforming entity in order to resolve the non conformity'*. If an audit revealed that a management procedure was not the latest edition, then a non conformity would exist. Replacement of the procedure with an up to date edition would dispose of the non conformity. However, there is also a need to find out why the situation existed, and for corrective action ('action taken to eliminate the causes of the existing non conformity or defect or other undesirable situation in order to prevent a recurrence'*) to be taken. For example, the situation described would require that a more secure system for document control be implemented.

The quality audit form used at St Elsewhere's is shown in Figure 11.12. The topic for audit is entered, together with the location, the auditors name and date of audit. A sequential number for the audit should be provided by the Quality Manager. In keeping with the numbering system used in St Elsewhere's Pathology laboratory, the first three digits represent the department. Number 000/14/96 would translate into the fourteenth audit in pathology in 1996 and 200/04/96 into the fourth audit in haematology in 1996. The next section on the form requires that details of all procedures, forms, records, etc. examined during the audit should be recorded. The record of non conformities follows and if there are no non conformities, it is important to record a nil value. In terms of prioritising the action to be taken when a non conformity is discovered, it is useful to categorise them as major or minor. The next step is to describe the steps required to dispose of the non conformity, and corrective action required to improve the situation, together with the timescale and name of the person responsible. The evidence that action has been taken and by whom should be recorded. This should be confirmed by the original auditor, and sent to the Quality Manager. If the reports raise important issues for the laboratory they can be discussed at the regular meetings of the QAU. The final step is to mark the form appropriately if issues have been identified during the course of a particular audit which might usefully be discussed at the next management review.

---

*ISO 8402:1994 Quality management and quality assurance-Vocabulary

St Elsewhere's Hospital Trust		QF 000 011
PATHOLOGY		**Edition1** **Page 1/2**

QUALITY AUDIT PROGRAMME
(MANAGEMENT PROCEDURES)

Year	*1996*

AUDIT TOPIC	Jan	Feb	Mar	Apr	May	Jun	Jul	Aug	Sep	Oct	Nov	Dec
Organisation & Management [MP 000 001]	3/1 ☒ JQ		3/1 CHECK ⟋ JQ						⟋			
Document preparation and control [MP 000 002]		3/1 ⟋ JQ							⟋			
Personnel management [MP 000 003]			3/1 ☒ JQ		CHECK ⟋							
Equipment Management [MP 000 004]				⟋						⟋		
Health and Safety [MP 000 005]				⟋								
Computer Management [MP 000 006]						⟋						
Purchasing Management [MP 000 007]						⟋						

PROGRESS IN THE QUALITY AUDIT PROGRAMME IS RECORDED AS SHOWN BELOW

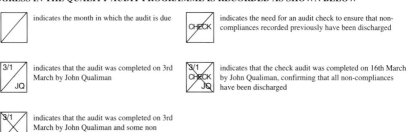

⟋	indicates the month in which the audit is due
CHECK ⟋	indicates the need for an audit check to ensure that non-compliances recorded previously have been discharged
3/1 ⟋ JQ	indicates that the audit was completed on 3rd March by John Qualiman
3/1 CHECK ⟋ JQ	indicates that the check audit was completed on 16th March by John Qualiman, confirming that all non-compliances have been discharged
3/1 ☒ JQ	indicates that the audit was completed on 3rd March by John Qualiman and some non compliances recorded

QUALITY FORM

Figure 11.11 Quality audit schedule (management procedures)

St Elsewhere's Hospital Trust	QF 000 012
	Edition1
PATHOLOGY	Page 1/1

QUALITY AUDIT FORM

AUDIT
ASPECT/ACTIVITY:-

LOCATION IN
LABORATORY:-   SERIAL NO:-

AUDITOR   DATE OF AUDIT

DETAILS OF PROCEDURES, FORMS/RECORDS, REPORTS EXAMINED DURING THE AUDIT

RECORD OF NON CONFORMITIES (please record nil where appropriate)   CATEGORY

ACTION REQUIRED (including timescale and person responsible)

ACTION COMPLETED BY (name)   ON (date)

CONFIRMED BY AUDITOR (name)   ON (date)

RECEIVED AND CONFIRMED BY QUALITY MANAGER (signature)   ON (date)

TO BE REFERRED TO THE NEXT MANAGEMENT REVIEW ON (date)

QUALITY FORM

Figure 11.12 Quality audit form

Most of the audit of management procedures refers to matters which can be done at a pathology laboratory level, and this may be true of certain laboratory procedures such as reception of samples. However, many audits of laboratory procedures may be delegated to particular departments. It is important when auditing laboratory procedures which describe methods of investigation or analysis to link them with the appropriate quality procedures for quality control and quality assessment. As in practice quality assessment and quality control is often peculiar to a discipline, it will be necessary to have separate procedures for each discipline. A similar approach can be taken to any clinical procedures, such as that for collecting blood specimens from patients, which may be a pathology responsibility or a departmental responsibility, commonly invested in the haematology department. Although delegation will take place, the quality manager should maintain overall control of the process.

In some texts quality audit is approached through horizontal audits or through vertical audits. If horizontal audit, say of equipment maintenance, is carried out only in a section of a department it may not reveal weaknesses in the way in which the quality system operates in that area. It is advisable to carry out an audit which goes across all departments and sections in pathology. An additional approach to the audit programme is to conduct vertical audits, in a sense to establish an audit trail through a particular procedure. This has been called process quality audit. However, when such audits are being conducted, it is likely that the distinction between different types of tools, quality audit, quality assessment, quality control and clinical audit may not be as important as addressing the issue which was raised.

In addition to the planned activity of auditing, which tends to be a 'top down' process, a system needs to be established in which queries can be raised about any aspect of departmental practice by any member of staff. Queries can include customer or staff complaints/criticisms/observations, problems with suppliers or goods received, or anything which is perceived to affect the quality of the laboratory's work. The query is then brought to the attention of a member of the QAU subcommittee who is responsible for completing a quality query form (Figure 11.13). The query itself must be clearly described and the initial response defined. A valid response is to take the query to the quality manager for presentation to the QAU subcommittee for discussion. The 'further action' section of the form must be completed and include the name of the person responsible for carrying out the action, and the specified time scale for such action. After the query has been dealt with, the query can be signed off, numbered and filed by the Quality Manager or, if it is seen to be of general importance, retained on the agenda of the QAU subcommittee for further discussion. However, some Quality Audit reports need to be referred to the Management review for further consideration.

St Elsewhere's Hospital Trust	QF 000 015
PATHOLOGY	Edition1 Page 1/1

QUALITY QUERY FORM

DATE OF QUERY:-

QAU subcommittee contact

QUERY FROM:-

SERIAL NO:-

ADDRESS

Telephone No.

QUERY

RESPONSE

ON (date)

RECEIVED AND CONFIRMED BY QUALITY MANAGER (signature)

ON (date)

TO BE REFERRED TO THE NEXT MANAGEMENT REVIEW ON (date)

QUALITY FORM

Figure 11.13 Quality query form

QUALITY ASSESSMENT/PROFICIENCY TESTING

The existence of quality assessment and proficiency testing has been one of the key factors in the improvement of pathology results. R J Maxwell, in his article on Quality assessment in health, said 'There are undoubtedly some outstanding examples of quality assessment activities in health services in Britain such as the confidential enquiry into maternal deaths, or the national quality control scheme in clinical chemistry' (as it was then called). In the same article he describes the scheme with commendable brevity. 'The scheme began in 1969. Every two weeks a portion of material is sent to all participating laboratories for analysis. They return their results of several commonly performed tests, and the data from all laboratories are compared. For each of the principal laboratory methods in use, the mean value, standard deviation, and variance index are calculated, thus each laboratory can compare its results to others while confidentiality is respected. Those who administer the scheme have been able to show progressive reduction in variance index, thus showing improvement in the consistency of results obtained by different laboratories.'

A useful definition of external quality assessment is given in Figure 11.14 and contrasting this with the definition of internal quality control from the same source (Figure 10.5) serves to reinforce their differing roles in quality assurance activities.

External quality assessment ...

'refers to a system of objectively checking laboratory results by means of an external agency. The checking is necessarily retrospective, and the comparison of a given laboratory's performance on a certain day with that of other laboratories cannot be notified to the laboratory until some time later. This comparison will not therefore have any influence on the tested laboratory's output on the day of the test. The main object of EQA is not to bring about day to day consistency but to establish between-laboratory comparability'

WHO External Assessment of Health Laboratories (1981)

Figure 11.14 Definition of external quality assessment

There is now an amazing diversity of schemes covering all disciplines of pathology. In many countries they were originally nurtured in the protective environment of the national health care schemes or in centres of academic excellence, but increasingly, excellent schemes have become available from commercial sources for the more routine assays. However the practical problems of setting up, for example, the UK scheme for breast screening pathology with its 300 UK participants, are of a magnitude greater than those of a general clinical chemistry with 600 participants. Even so, obtaining material which is commutable with human samples still poses problems in clinical chemistry.

In many schemes there are advantages of participation that go beyond the ability to compare the performance of one's own laboratory against overall performance of other laboratories. Schemes which deal with quantitative assays will subdivide the participants into method groups or into instrumentation groups, and this enables the participant to judge whether they are 'running with the tide' or whether they stand in splendid isolation and still use Folin and Wu's technique for blood sugar assays. This data informs the laboratory on trends in different methods of measurement, for example the change from gas chromato- graphic techniques to fluorescent polarisation or enzyme mediated immunoassays in therapeutic drug monitoring. A further important aspect of EQA is the use of schemes for broader educational purposes. For example, the scheme organiser will not only send out samples for analysis but will devise a clinical context within which the results have to be interpreted. This approach brings into play not only the ability of a laboratory to produce accurate results but also requires that they be interpreted against the laboratory's reference values and in the context of a clinical question.

Standard F2 of CPA(UK)Ltd stresses the importance not only of belonging to schemes but also that 'Where appropriate, quality assessment programmes are widely publicised in the department with regular formal review of performance'. The guideline to the standard states 'the results of internal quality control and external quality assessment programmes should be presented in such a way that they are readily available to and understood by all members of the section in which the analytical work is done'. This requirement should be seen as an essential part of the continuous training of all laboratory staff.

RELATIONSHIP TO ACCREDITATION

Accreditation schemes designed for pathology laboratories such as CAP-LAP and CPA(UK)Ltd require participation in recognised quality assessment or proficiency testing schemes. The schemes themselves, and the laboratory's performance in the schemes, have not only become an integral part of the accreditation process but in many countries the determinant of whether the laboratory can continue to operate or get reimbursed for their work. The relationship between a particular accreditation system and participation in an external quality assessment scheme varies from the CAP-LAP situation where it is a requirement that the laboratory participates in CAP proficiency testing schemes, to CPA(UK)Ltd which requires that 'The department must subscribe to approved External Quality Assessment Schemes corresponding to their repertoire' and to accreditation sys- tems which mandate participation in particular schemes at certain times. These schemes can be run by commercial concerns, universities, or by non profit making organisations such as the Canadian Reference Foundation/Fondation Canadienne de Référence which is currently mandated by the provinces of British Columbia and Alberta to provide external quality assessment schemes in general chemistry and lipids.

The emerging situation in the United Kingdom is of particular interest. CPA (UK) Ltd. was originally set up to undertake the accreditation of laboratories, but as can be seen in Figure 11.15 there are now two distinct parts of CPA(UK)Ltd both reporting to the management board. The original task (activity A_1) of CPA(UK)Ltd was accrediting clinical pathology laboratories and is shown on the left. How that operates will be discussed in Chapter 12, The Inspector calls. The side labelled A_2 is responsible for accrediting external quality assessment schemes, and advice is given to the board by a multidisciplinary CPA(EQA) advisory committee. When a laboratory applies for accreditation it undertakes two commitments with regard to quality assessment. One states 'application for accreditation should be made only by departments willing to allow its performance in external quality assessment schemes to be made known to CPA', and the other involves ticking a box on

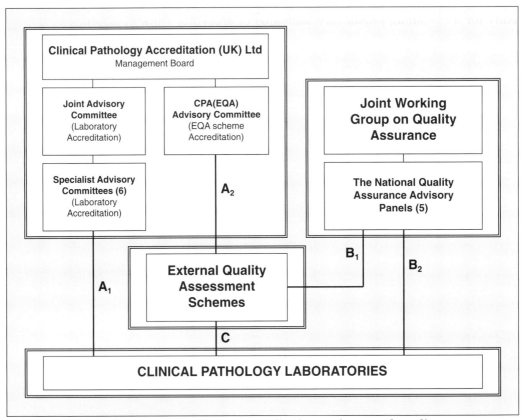

Figure 11.15 The relationship between accreditation and external quality assessment in the United Kingdom.

the application form to indicate whether in the past two years, there has been any persistent poor performance in any External Quality Assessment Scheme. Details should be sent with the application form if there has been persistent poor performance. The purpose of requiring details is not only that the nature of the poor performance is described but that the response to the poor performance is documented. Accreditation of external assessment schemes is discussed in the next section.

The monitoring of a laboratory's performance in quality assessment or proficiency testing schemes is the responsibility of a separate independent body, the Joint Working Group on Quality Assurance (JWGQA), shown on the right of Figure 11.15. Both this group and the National Quality Assurance Advisory Panels (NQAAP) consist of representatives of professional bodies concerned with pathology. The responsibility of JWGQA on behalf of its professional bodies is to monitor and support the NQAAP (Panels) particularly in their relationships with laboratories and quality assessment scheme organisers. It is a professional 'watchdog', independent of government. The Panels themselves have the responsibility for maintaining satisfactory standards of analytical work in laboratories (Figure 11.15, activity B_1) and do this by working closely with the organisers of quality assessment schemes. The EQA organisers bring to the attention of the appropriate Panel any laboratory whose performance and/or frequency of returns are judged to be unsatisfactory by criteria agreed by the Panels with the appropriate steering committees. At this preliminary stage the laboratories are only known to the Panels by a code number. If the Panel, on considering the information, feels it appropriate to intervene then a 'Dear Colleague' letter goes via the organiser to the laboratory to ask about the problem and offer support and advice. If the participating laboratory does not respond and the problems continue, then the chairman of the panel will obtain the address of the laboratory from the scheme organiser and communicate directly with the head of the department to seek a resolution (Figure 11.15, activity B_2).

Thus the process of accreditation and monitoring performance in external assessment schemes are separate. The only connection between the NQAAP and CPA(UK)Ltd is that the chairmen of the panels are co-opted members of the CPA special advisory committees for liaison purposes. This 'voluntary' system of participation in external quality assessment is in marked contrast to the situation in other parts of Europe such as Germany, where legislation requires that quality assessment of quantitative analyses in medical laboratories is prescribed in accordance with the guidelines of the Federal Medical Association. In the United States under the final requirements of CLIA'88 for proficiency testing, target values are set for the majority of analytes and laboratories are classified as either successful, probation, or suspended, which seem to be self explanatory terms! For each analyte on three occasions a year the laboratory analyses five samples and must measure four out of five correctly, that is within the allowable error of the reference value. By standards in other countries this is a very low exposure to quality assessment there are an increasing number of critics arguing that this may not be the most effective way of securing an environment in which a continuous improvement of quality can take place and they look to less regulation and a more informed approach to quality assessment.

ACCREDITATION OF QUALITY ASSESSMENT PROGRAMMES
When an accreditation body makes a statement to the effect that laboratories must participate in approved external assessment schemes, then it raises the issue of what is to be

considered as an approved scheme. ISO/IEC Guide No.43-1984(E) which is entitled 'Development and operation of laboratory proficiency testing', has three objectives:

- to assist in the selection and organisation of interlaboratory test comparisons for proficiency testing

- to describe the factors which should be taken into account in proficiency testing

- to describe how bodies assessing the technical competence of testing laboratories may use proficiency testing.

Interlaboratory test comparisons are defined as the 'organisation, performance and evaluations of tests on the same or similar items or materials by two or more different laboratories in accordance with predetermined conditions'. In the UK the Joint Working Party on Quality Assurance have produced some useful criteria to use in assessing external quality assessment schemes and, as described earlier, CPA(UK)Ltd has been given the task of accrediting EQA schemes in the UK and is developing standards based on the criteria in ISO/IEC Guide No.43-1984(E), cross referencing them with the ISO 9000 series of standards. The CPA(UK)Ltd standards are in two sections. The standards in the first part are in sections as shown in Figure 11.16. The second section concerns aspects of the organisations providing schemes. In Australia, NPAAC has published an important series of volumes entitled 'Criteria for the Assessment of External Quality Assurance Programs', see Further Reading for details.

---

1. Organisation, direction and administration of schemes

2. EQA scheme design and performance analysis

3. Communications with participants in EQA schemes

4. Manufacture of EQA material

5. Evaluation of EQA schemes

Figure 11.16 Sections of standards for external quality assessment schemes (EQA)

CLINICAL AUDIT

Although Clinical or Medical Audit may be thought of as a recent innovation, Florence Nightingale in a methodical assessment of the standards of medical care in Army hospitals in the Crimea showed that 'the key determinant of regimental mortality was distance from hospital. The least fortunate regiments were those with good access to hospital beds, because deaths depended less on casualties in battle than on acquiring an infection in hospital', an excellent example of clinical audit which has its echoes in the modern day problems with Methicillin resistant *Staphylococcus aureus*.

It is salutary to realise that as long ago as 1919, 'The Minimum Standard' promulgated by the American College of Surgeons of North America (described in Chapter 1), included in Section 4 a description of doctors organising themselves as a professional body and conducting medical audit on a regular basis (Figure 11.17). Audit conducted by doctors alone is termed medical audit, but when the work is undertaken on a multidisciplinary basis it is termed clinical audit. Health care outcome, as we saw in the discussion of quality in Chapter 2, is used to denote a change in a patient's current and future health status as a result of a particular intervention, such as a course of treatment or the performance of a surgical procedure.

In that the staff initiate and, with the approval of the governing board of the hospital, adopt rules, regulations, and policies governing the professional work of the hospital; that these rules, regulations, and policies specifically provide:-

(a) That staff meetings be held at least once each month. (In large hospitals the departments may chose to meet separately).

(b) That the staff review and analyze at regular intervals their clinical experience in the various departments of the hospital, such as medicine, surgery, obstetrics, and the other specialities; the clinical records of patients, free and pay, to be the basis for such review and analyses.

Figure 11.17 Section 4 of The Minimum Standard

A number of different definitions have been given of clinical audit, three of which are shown in Figure 11.18 All the definitions have a slightly different emphasis but the key issues are a systematic and critical approach, the involvement of all appropriate staff, and focus on patient care. As it is conducted in a cyclical manner, there is a continuing process of evaluation which it is intended should lead to the maintenance or improvement in clinical effectiveness.

As the timeliness, accuracy and appropriateness of preanalytical, analytical and postanalytical process activities can have a profound effect on patient treatment, audit of these aspects of operating process activities can be considered a clinical audit. The performance of a laboratory in external quality assessment schemes might be regarded as a surrogate for performance on a patient specimen, but any clinical audit must encompass broader issues such as evaluating the choice of test or procedure in the context of diagnosis, prognosis or monitoring of disease, and whether it had an appropriate effect on the healthcare outcome for an individual patient. In comparison with the rather mechanical nature of the quality audits described earlier, clinical audit should be seen as an opportunity to develop innovative approaches to ensuring and assuring quality in patient care.

Clinical audit...

'...involves systematically looking at procedures used for the diagnosis, care and treatment, examining how associated resources are used and investigating the effect care has on the outcome and quality of life for the patient'

UK Department of Health (1993)

'...is a process in which doctors, nurses and other health care professionals systematically review, and where necessary make changes to, the care and treatment they provide to patients. Its primary objective is to improve the quality and outcome of patient care'

Clinical Audit in England (1995) National Audit Office

'...is colleagues reflecting on their work systematically, critically and openly, to enable them to agree how to do it better and check improvements occur'

John Gabbay (1993) Wessex Institute of Public Health Medicine

Figure 11.18 Definitions of clinical audit

THE CLINICAL AUDIT CYCLE

An audit cycle spiral is not unfamiliar in the context of quality audit where the process of audit can result in the identification of non conformances which in turn may result in a need for change. Figure 11.19 shows the steps in the clinical audit cycle and although this is not a text on how to carry out clinical audit, brief explanation will lead into some of the activities in which pathology laboratories can participate. The first step is the identification of an issue or topic for audit, such as,

- Why are inadequate smears for cervical cytology received from a particular general practice?

- Is the correct action taken when a patient is found to have a low sodium or a high potassium?

- Does the laboratory follow up a high mean cell volume with appropriate tests?

- Are cardiac markers useful in the management of suspected myocardial infarction?

or perhaps the universal issue of turnaround time. The next step is to determine the purpose and nature of the service required and perform a literature search to see if there is any previous work on the topic. Then follows the negotiation of an agreed procedure and determination of the objective criteria against which practice can be measured.

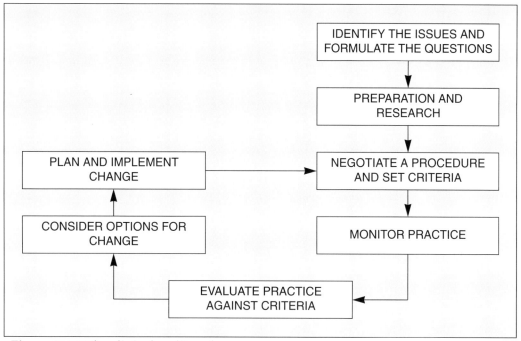

Figure 11.19 The clinical audit cycle

After monitoring practice, an evaluation takes place. If the criteria have not been met, options for change have to be considered and a plan made to implement the change. If necessary the procedure is then renegotiated and the cycle repeated. Implementation of change is crucial if improvements in outcome are to be effected. To be effective implementation of change should come about through education rather than by management dictate.

OPPORTUNITIES FOR CLINICAL AUDIT

Clinical audit creates the opportunity for all laboratory staff to understand their individual contribution to the well-being of patients. This can be an important factor in motivating staff to perform well. It was the practice many years ago, and may still exist in some centres, for technical staff to go out and collect blood samples from the hospital wards. This practice has now been largely superseded by the advent of phlebotomists which may appear to be a more effective use of staff, but reduces the opportunity for staff to see and understand the situation of the patients.

It is important to understand that clinical audit offers the opportunity for interface between the laboratory discipline and a clinical speciality, and Figure 11.20 gives some ideas for those involved in this interface and the issues which might be identified as topics suitable for audit. Once the question 'What does the doctor/patient require? has been asked, it should be difficult to stop the ideas coming.

Laboratory discipline	Clinical speciality	Issues and questions
Biochemistry	Cardiology	Would speedy return of digoxin and cardiac marker results improve clinical management?
	Diabetology	Should the annual review of patients with diabetes include a microalbumin assay?
	General Practice	Is the interpretation of PSA results helpful?
	Neurology	Are sodium valproate levels of any value?
	Accident and emergency	Would it be useful to have a blood gas analyser in Accident and Emergency maintained by the laboratory?
Haematology	Anaesthetics and surgery	Are the guidelines for the use of blood and blood products working effectively?
	Medicine	Formulate guidelines for the use of anticoagulants
	General Practice	Are requests for vitamin B12 and red cell folate useful?
Microbiology	Whole hospital	Infection control
	General Practice	Review procedure for collection and transportation of samples
	Paediatrics	Review policy on diagnosis of urinary tract infection
Histopathology	Gastroenterology	Detection and monitoring of coeliac disease
	Clinical Biochemistry	Evaluate PSA results with histological investigation of the prostate
	Surgery	Audit post mortems on post operative deaths
	Gynaecology	Do colposcopy findings correlate with histology and cytology findings?

Figure 11.20 Issues and topics for clinical audit

Figure 11.21 gives further areas for clinical audit in relation to the different steps in operating process activities. In each discipline of pathology it should be possible to identify many different areas of legitimate concern. If possible the execution of the audit should be done in a way which enables repeat audits to be performed with the minimum of effort. For example, in relation to the timeliness of the service, many pathology computers can give turnaround times from the time of logging the specimen on the computer (which is not the same as when it arrived in the laboratory) to printing or transmission of the report. However, timeliness may be more important as a measure of the time from which the specimen is collected (from the patient) until the requesting doctor receives the report, and conducting such a audit is a more complex and time consuming exercise.

Finally, perhaps the most important topic for clinical research and audit is to ascertain whether the work which has been done to determine the usefulness of diagnostic tests is well founded. An extremely important review article entitled 'Use of Methodological

Steps in the operating process activities	Areas for audit
1. Doctor/patient consultation	Are request cards suitably designed and readily available?
2. Request form completed	Are adequate clinical details provided?
3. Specimen collection	Does the Users handbook contain satisfactory information?
4. Specimen and request form transportation	Are the model rules available for the personnel involved in transporting specimens?
5. Specimen and request form reception	Is a check made to ensure that the specimen container details agree with the request card details?
6. Data acquisition from specimen and request form	Are clinical details entered into the computer accurately?
7. Specimen preparation	Is the specimen received appropriate for the investigation required?
8. Specimen analysis	Has agreement been reached on which tests are appropriate for the clinical condition being investigated?
9. Reporting of results including interpretation and recommendations	Does the report contain a satisfactory interpretative comment where required?
10. Transmission of report	Is the turnaround time for results appropriate for the clinical situation under investigation?
11. Receipt of report by the doctor, and consultation as appropriate	Is adequate interpretative advice available twenty four hours per day?

Figure 11.21 Issues for audit in relation to operating process activity

Standards in Diagnostic Test Research' (see Further Reading) concluded 'that most diagnostic tests are still inadequately appraised' and suggests that 'The routine demand for methodological standards could raise the quality of diagnostic test information, and the careful predissemination evaluation of diagnostic tests could eliminate useless tests before they receive widespread application.'

PROCEDURE FOR THE MANAGEMENT OF QUALITY ASSURANCE

Figure 11.22 gives the contents of a procedure for the management of quality assurance. This procedure should be regarded as a 'framework' procedure to which other quality procedures can be referenced.

Content of procedure

1.0   Purpose and Scope

2.0   Responsibility

3.0   References

4.0   Definitions

5.0   Documentation

6.0   Action and methods

    6.1 Management responsibilities
       6.1.1 The Quality Policy
       6.1.2 Management representative (Quality Manager)
       6.1.3 Management review

    6.2 The Quality Assurance Unit subcommittee
       6.2.1 Chairperson, deputy chairperson and secretary
       6.2.2 Membership and co-option
       6.2.3 Responsibilities of members
       6.2.4 Departmental quality groups

    6.3 Departmental quality groups
       6.3.1 Quality Assessment/Quality control review
       6.3.2 Clinical Audit reports
       6.3.3 Delegated Quality Audit

    6.4 Frequency of meetings
       6.4.1 Quality Assurance Unit subcommittee
       6.4.2 Department Quality groups

    6.5 Agenda of meetings
       6.5.1 Attendance
       6.5.2 Minutes of previous meeting
       6.5.3 Progress report on current quality plan
       6.5.4 Quality Audit Review
       6.5.5 Reports from Departmental quality groups
          • Quality Assessment/Quality control reviews
          • Clinical Audit reports
       6.5.6 Preparation for Management review
       6.5.7 Any other business

    6.6 Minutes of meetings
       6.6.1 Format and numbering
       6.6.2 Distribution

    6.7 Communications
       6.7.1 Quality Audit Review
       6.7.2 Minutes of the QAU sub committee
       6.7.3 Management review

Figure 11.22 Content of a procedure for management of quality assurance

REQUIREMENTS FOR QUALITY ASSURANCE

The requirements of different quality and accreditation systems in relation to quality assurance are shown in Figure 11.23.

System	Quality assurance and quality control

ISO 9001:1994	**4. Quality system requirements** *(see Figure 11.6)*
	4.1 Management responsibility
	    4.1.1 *Quality policy*
	    4.1.2 *Organisation*
	    4.1.3 *Management review*
	4.2 Quality system.
	    4.2.1 *General*
	    4.2.2 *Quality system procedures*
	    4.2.3 *Quality planning*
	4.5 Document and data control *(see Chapter 4)*
	    4.5.1 *General*
	    4.5.2 *Document and data approval and issue*
	    4.5.3 *Document and data changes*
	4.14 Corrective and preventative action
	    4.14.1 *General*
	    4.14.2 *Corrective action*
	    4.14.3 *Preventative action*
	4.17 Internal quality audits

EN 45001:1989	**5 Technical competence** **5.4 Working procedures** **5.4.2** *Quality Systems* The laboratory shall operate a Quality System appropriate to the type, range and volume of work performed. The elements of this system shall be documented in a Quality Manual which is available for use by the laboratory personnel… A person or persons having responsibility for quality assurance within the laboratory shall be designated by laboratory management and have direct access to top management… The quality system shall be systematically and periodically reviewed by or on behalf of management to ensure the continued effectiveness of the arrangements, and any necessary corrective action initiated. Such reviews shall be recorded together with details of any corrective action taken.
OECD - GLP	**1. Test facility organisation and personnel** **1.1 Management's responsibilities** (2) at a minimum it should: (f) ensure that there is a Quality Assurance Programme with designated personnel **2. Quality Assurance Programme** **2.1 General** (1) The test facility should have a documented quality assurance programme to ensure that studies performed are in compliance with these Principles of Good Laboratory Practice. (2) The quality assurance programme should be carried out by an individual or by individuals designated by and directly responsible to management and who are familiar with the test procedures. (3) This individual(s) should not be involved in the conduct of the study being assured. (4) This individual(s) should report any findings in writing directly to management and to the Study Director.

	2.2 Responsibilities of the Quality Assurance Personnel
	(1) The responsibilities of the quality assurance personnel should include, but not be limited to, the following functions:
	    (a) Ascertain that the study plan and Standard Operating procedures are available to personnel conducting the study;
	    (b) Ensure that the study plan and Standard Operating Procedures are followed by periodic inspections of the test facility and/or by auditing the study in progress. Records of such procedures should be retained;
	    (c) Promptly report to management and the Study Director unauthorised deviations from the study plan and from Standard Operating Procedures;
	    (d) Review the final reports to confirm that the methods, procedures, and observations are accurately described, and that the reported results accurately reflect the raw data of the study;
	    (e) Prepare and sign a statement, to be included with the final report, which specifies the dates inspections were made and the dates any findings were reported to management and to the Study Director.

CAP - LAP	**Standard III Quality assurance** There shall be an ongoing quality assurance program designed to monitor and evaluate objectively and systematically the quality and appropriateness of the care and treatment provided to patients by the pathology service, to pursue opportunities to patients by the pathology service, and to identify and resolve problems. **Standard IV Quality control** Each pathology service shall have a quality control system that demonstrates the reliability and medical usefulness of laboratory data.
CPA(UK)Ltd	**F Evaluation** **F1.** The department must have a formal policy for internal quality control and must participate in recognised external quality assessment programmes. **F2.** Where appropriate quality assessment programmes are widely publicised in the department with regular formal review of performance. **F3.** Quality assurance evaluation includes continuing clinical audit of the service provided. **F4.** Senior pathology staff participate in audit activities with other clinical specialities

Figure 11.23 Requirements for quality assurance

FURTHER READING

Campbell F, Griffiths D F R. Quantitative audit of the content of histopathology reports, J Clin Pathol 1994;**47**:360-361.

Carrington Reid M, Lachs M S, Feinstein A R. Use of Methodological Standards in Diagnostic Test Research: Getting Better but Still Not Good 1995; **274**:546-651.

Castaneda-Mendez K. Proficiency Testing from a total quality management perspective, Clin Chem 1992; **38**:615-618.

Clinical Audit in England, 1995, National Audit Office HC 27 HMSO.

Clinical Audit in Pathology, June 1995, The Royal College of Pathologists UK.

Criteria for the Assessment of External Quality Assurance Programs,

Vol.1, Clinical Biochemistry, Haematology, Microbiology 1995.

Vol.2, Transfusion Serology, Anatomical Pathology, and Cytology 1996.

Commonwealth Department of Health (Australia), National Pathology Accreditation Advisory Council.

Donabedian A. Evaluating the Quality of Medical Care, Millbank Memorial Fund Quarterly 1996; **44**:166-206.

External Quality Assessment of Health Laboratories (1979), EURO Reports and Studies 36, World Health Organization.

Good Laboratory Practice and the role of quality assurance, Advisory Leaflet No.3, (1991) United Kingdom GLP Compliance Programme, Department of Health, London.

Guidelines for post mortem reports (1993), The Royal College of Pathologists London UK.

ISO 8402:1994, Quality management and quality assurance - Vocabulary.

Maxwell R J. Quality Assessment in Health, 1984; BMJ **288**:1470-1472.

Moore A, Muir Gray J A, McQuay, H. How good is that Test? Bandolier 1996; 3:1-3.

Nomenclature and Definitions For Use in NRSCL and other NCCLS Documents, Second Edition (1993), NCCLS Proposed Guideline NRSCL8-P2, Vol.13, No.1.

Olazabal D A V R. Guidelines for the Organization of National Quality Assessment Programmes, LAB/83.11, World Health Organization.

Practice Protocol for the Examination of Specimens Removed from Patients with Carcinoma of the Prostate Gland, Arch Path and Lab Med, 1994, CAP Document B266.

Platt S F. Establishing one quality assurance system to meet the requirements of ISO 9001, NAMAS and GLP. The VAM Bulletin 1993; **9**, 7-10.

Quality Assurance for Commercially Prepared Microbiological Culture Media; Approved Standard (1990). NCCLS Document M22-A.

Quality Audit and Quality System Review in Calibration and Testing Laboratories, 1991. NAMAS Executive Document M51.

Reid M C, Lacks M S, and Feinstein A R. Use of methodological standards in diagnostic test research-getting better but still not good. JAMA 1995; **274**:645-651.

Standards in Infection Control in Hospitals (1993) Association of Medical Microbiologists, Hospital Infection Society, Infection Control Nurses Association, Public Health Laboratory Service.

The Autopsy and Audit, Report of the Joint Working Party of the Royal College of Pathologists, the Royal College of Physicians of London and the Royal College of Surgeons of England (1991).

The Evolution of Clinical Audit 1995, The Department of Health UK.

The Quality Manual, Guidance for Preparation M16, (1996) NAMAS, United Kingdom Accreditation Service.

Thompson M, Wood R. International Harmonized Protocol for Proficiency Testing of (Chemical) Analytical Laboratories, 1993; J of AOAC International **76**:926-937.

Chapter 12

The Inspector calls...

INTRODUCTION

In order to gain recognition as being compliant with a particular quality or accreditation system it is necessary for the laboratory to go through an inspection process. This process can usefully be examined in three phases, preinspection, inspection and postinspection. This chapter will discuss and look at:

- authority for accreditation and certification
- standards for accreditation and certification bodies
- requirements for accreditation
- the process involved in an inspection
- the selection and training of inspectors

and finally will have a brief look at the changing scene and the way ahead. The author's preference is for a less regulatory sounding term than inspector, but as the term is in general use it will be used in this chapter. Other terms used include audit/auditor, assessment/assessor and survey/surveyor.

AUTHORITY FOR ACCREDITATION AND CERTIFICATION

In Chapter 2 it was indicated that EN 45001:1989 is one of a series of standards which not only indicate the general criteria for operation of a testing laboratory (EN 45001), but also give general criteria for the assessment of laboratories (EN 45002) and for laboratory accreditation bodies (EN 45003). As similar arrangements are emerging in different European countries for accreditation and certification activities, the United Kingdom (UK) can be illustrative of the general case. In the UK the United Kingdom Accreditation Service (UKAS) is the body concerned with accreditation of laboratories and certification bodies (Figure 12.1). Its recognition as the sole body to carry out these activities derives from a memorandum of understanding between UKAS and the Secretary of State for Trade and Industry in the UK Government. It records a joint commitment to maintaining and developing a strong and unified national accreditation service in the UK and sees it as a means of promoting the quality and competitiveness of UK industry. Similar arrangements exist in other European Countries. As can be seen from Figure 12.1, UKAS has direct authority to accredit laboratories to EN 45001. Whereas in Sweden experience with EN 45001 standards in pathology is quite extensive, in the UK experience is limited to a few pathology laboratories. UKAS also accredits certification bodies which in turn can inspect organisations (including laboratories), for compliance with the ISO 9000 series of standards. A Haematology laboratory in Plymouth UK has recognition with respect to BS 5750 (equivalent to BS EN ISO 9000 series) and has been generous in sharing that experience with the author.

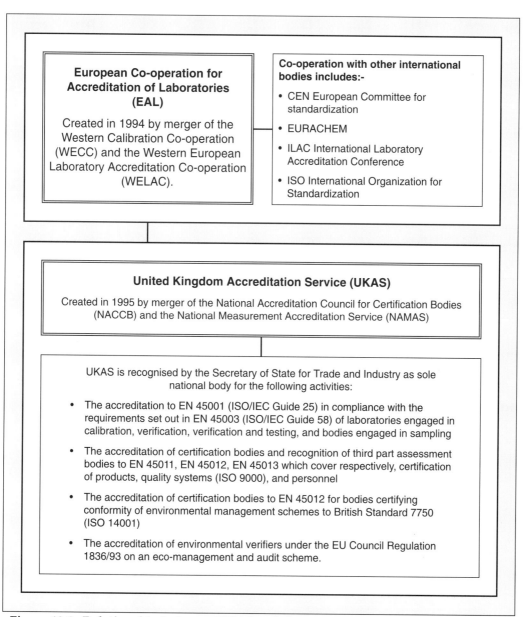

Figure 12.1 Relationship between UKAS and the EAL

With respect to the accreditation of laboratories, UKAS in turn belongs to the European Co-operation for Accreditation of Laboratories (EAL) and co-operates with other international bodies directly and in concert with EAL. The prime objective of EAL is 'the immediate and unquestioned acceptance of accredited test reports and calibration certificates throughout Europe and eventually throughout the world.' All EAL member bodies must 'satisfy themselves fully that each of their members individually is operating in full compliance with EN 45002 and EN 45003 and/or the equivalent ISO/IEC Guide 58.' This then enables them to deduce that test reports and calibration certificates issued by accredited laboratories conform to EN 45001 and are mutually acceptable. In addition to this arrangement national accreditation bodies negotiate bilateral or multilateral mutual recognition agreements with other countries.

CAP-LAP has authority for its accreditation activities in the USA by virtue both of its pioneering activity in the field of accreditation and the fact that it is a deemed status in relation to CLIA'88 legislation. In contrast CPA(UK)Ltd, which now has the practical experience of inspecting in excess of eight hundred departments of laboratories in the UK and one in Italy, is not formally recognised by the UK Government. Unlike a number of European countries there is no legislation governing the conduct of clinical pathology in the UK. However a recent NHS Executive report entitled 'Strategic Review of Pathology Services', contains a chapter on 'Service Quality' in which the role of accreditation is mentioned with particular reference to CPA(UK)Ltd. After discussing the potential benefits of accreditation to both the providers and purchasers of pathology services, it concludes 'We recommend that purchasers and providers incorporate accreditation or a commitment to obtain accreditation as a condition of any pathology contract'.

With respect to monitoring compliance with 'The Principles of GLP', different countries make their own individual arrangements but seek bilateral and multilateral recognition agreements. In the UK, for example, a GLP Monitoring Unit was established in 1983 in the Department of Health and Social Security (now the Department of Health). Its inspections fall into two distinct categories. The first is a regular monitoring of laboratories, normally on a biannual basis and the second, at the request of a regulatory authority in the UK or abroad, to perform study audits which occasionally also involve laboratory inspections. It is for the requesting regulatory authority to justify the need for such inspections or audits. In order to meet international requirements, inspections and audits are conducted in accordance with the OECD Principles of GLP and they are also in conformity with the EEC directives, 87/18/EEC, 'on harmonization of laws, regulations and administrative provisions relating to the application of the principles of good laboratory practice and the verification of their applications for tests on chemical substances' (and 88/320/EEC 'on the inspection and verification of Good Laboratory Practice (GLP)'. Although there are differences in the different codes there is now a Memorandum of

---

*OJ No L 15/29 17th January 1987 and OJ No L 145/35 11th June 1988

Understanding for mutual recognition of the Principles of GLP promulgated by the OECD, the US Food and Drug Administration (FDA) and the US Environmental Protection Agency (EPA).

STANDARDS FOR ACCREDITATION AND CERTIFICATION BODIES

In Europe, EAL requires that member bodies operate in accord with the criteria of EN 45003:1989 the standard for bodies accrediting laboratories, and also apply the criteria of EN 45011-13 in their role of accrediting certifying bodies. The criteria for laboratory accreditation bodies given in EN 45003:1989 have many similarities to those for the accreditation of certification bodies (EN 45011-13), and Figure 12.2 compares the contents of each system using the example of EN 45003 and 45012.

EN 45012:1989 General Criteria for certification bodies operating quality system certification	EN 45003:1989 General criteria for laboratory accreditation bodies
1. Object and field of application	1. Object and field of application
2. Definitions	2. Definitions
3. General requirements	3. General requirements
4. Administrative structure	4. Organisation
5. Terms of reference of governing board	5. Personnel and impartial experts
	6. Policy and decision making process
6. Organizational structure	7. Sectoral committees
7. Certification personnel	5. Personnel and impartial experts
8. Documentation and change control	
9. Records	15. Records
10. Certification and surveillance procedures	9. Arrangements for accreditation
11. Certification and surveillance facilities required	9. Arrangements for accreditation
12. Quality Manual	8. Quality system
13. Confidentiality	13. Confidentiality
14. Publications	14. Publications
15. Appeals	11. Appeals procedure
16. Internal audit and periodic review	8. Quality system
17. Misuse of certificates	10. Accreditation documents
18. Complaints	9. Arrangements for accreditation
19. Withdrawal and cancellation of certificates	9. Arrangements for accreditation
	12. Contractual arrangements
	16. Delegation
	17. Exchange of experience

Figure 12.2   Contents of EN 45012/EN 45003 compared

The other form of accreditation of relevance to laboratories is the accreditation of proficiency schemes (external quality schemes) and, whereas ISO/IEC guide 34:1984 does not give criteria for the body carrying out the accreditation, it does define the criteria for the development and operation of laboratory proficiency testing.

REQUIREMENTS FOR INSPECTION

In the case of CAP-LAP and EN 45001:1989, the inspection requirements form part of the actual standard and these two situations will be described in some detail to indicate the features that are common to the inspection process. Figure 12.3 gives the requirements contained in the CAP-LAP Standard V. The first paragraph of the interpretative notes outline the preinspection requirements, and the second the requirement for the inspection. The last paragraph outlines the circumstances when the direction or ownership changes and the post inspection requirement for periodic self evaluation.

STANDARD V INSPECTION REQUIREMENTS

A pathology service that desires accreditation shall undergo periodic inspections and evaluations as determined by the Commission on Laboratory Accreditation of the College of American Pathologists

INTERPRETATION

The applicant process will be initiated by the submission of a completed application containing the necessary information, evidence of enrolment in the appropriate proficiency testing programs, and payment of fees. Laboratories will be evaluated in accordance with the Standards for Laboratory Accreditation of the College of American Pathologists.

The pathology service must submit to a complete periodic on-site inspection. The Commission will not inspect or accredit a portion of a single cohesive laboratory except under special and/or unusual circumstances, and then only by prior arrangements with, or approval of, the Regional Commissioner. The conduct of inspections and evaluation of results shall be in accordance with the policies and procedures of the Commission on Laboratory Accreditation.

Laboratories undergoing a change in directorship, location, or ownership are subject to inspection and evaluation in accordance with applicable policy.

Laboratories enrolled in the Laboratory Accreditation Program are required to perform periodic self-evaluations. When deficiencies are noted, the laboratory shall take appropriate corrective action, which shall be documented and subject to review by the Commission on Laboratory Accreditation. Uncorrected deficiencies at the next on-site inspection shall be considered recurrent. The Commissioner(s) will review deficiencies detected during self-evaluation. Corrective action responses from the laboratory director may be required

Recurrence of the same deficiencies in consecutive inspections is considered a serious problem and is subject to review by the Commission

---

Figure 12.3 CAP-LAP Standard V Inspection Requirements

The EN 45001:1989 system also has requirements for inspection written in the standard and section 6.2 Co-operation with bodies granting accreditation is shown in Figure 12.4 which in essence contains many of the features of the CAP-LAP and other systems.

A further item that is included in Section 7 of EN 45001:1989 details duties resulting from accreditation. These duties consist of continuing at all times to comply with the requirements of the standard and with criteria prescribed by the body which actually grants accreditation, making the claim for accreditation, paying appropriate fees to the body granting accreditation, not using accreditation in such a way that brings the granting body into disrepute, and upon termination of accreditation discontinuing the claim to being accredited in all advertising material.

Co-operation with bodies granting accreditation

The testing laboratory shall afford the body granting accreditation and its representative such reasonable co-operation as is necessary, to enable the body granting accreditation to monitor compliance with these requirements and other criteria. This co-operation shall include:

a) affording the representative access to relevant areas of the testing laboratory, for the witnessing of tests;

b) undertaking any reasonable check to enable the body granting accreditation to verify the testing capability of the testing laboratory;

c) preparation, packaging and dispatch of test samples or items needed by the body granting accreditation for verification purposes;

d) participation in any appropriate programme of proficiency testing or comparison testing that the body granting accreditation may reasonably deem to be necessary;

e) permitting scrutiny by the body granting accreditation of the results of the testing laboratory's own internal audits or proficiency tests.

Figure 12.4 EN 45001:1989 Co-operation with bodies granting accreditation

It also requires that all contracts made with clients should state that the fact that accreditation has been granted does not constitute product approval by that body. There is also a requirement to ensure that no test report used by a client shall be used for promotion or publicity purposes if the body granting accreditation feels that this might be misleading. No test report should be reproduced by the client, in full or in part for promotional or publicity purposes, without written approval of both the body granting accreditation and the testing laboratory. Finally there is a requirement to inform immediately the body granting accreditation of any changes which might affect the laboratory's status as an accredited laboratory.

For a national organisation like UKAS which carries out the accreditation of laboratories according to the EN 45001:1989 standard, the standard EN 45002 gives the general criteria to be followed in assessing laboratories. In this standard the accreditation process is described as the gathering of information needed for the evaluation of an applicant laboratory, the appointment of one or more qualified assessor, the on site assessment and the review of evaluation material collected. This is followed by a decision to grant accreditation, with or without conditions, or to refuse accreditation to the applicant laboratory. The definition of the scope or activities of the laboratory forms part of the certificate of accreditation. In common with other systems mention is made of an appeal mechanism, 'Any decision to refuse or limit the scope of accreditation shall be taken after the laboratory concerned has had the possibility of a hearing'. EN 45002 includes ongoing surveillance at regular intervals regarding five years as the maximum interval before a repeat assessment takes place. Figure 12.5 shows the stages used by UKAS. The steps described above are very similar to those used in any accreditation or certification process.

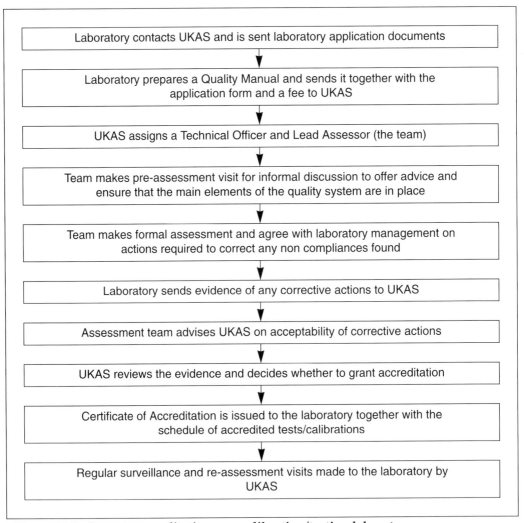

Figure 12.5 Steps to accreditation as a calibration/testing laboratory

INSPECTION

In the sections which follow the material is mainly drawn from the experience of the CAP-LAP and CPA(UK)Ltd systems which are specific to clinical pathology laboratories. Much of the content will be mirrored in other systems operating in different parts of the world, such as Canada and Australia, and is not dissimilar from the approach used by more generic quality and accreditation systems.

PREINSPECTION

The CAP-LAP process is described in greater detail in the 'Laboratory Accreditation Manual' (see Further Reading), and what follows is a brief summary. In the preinspection phase, stress is laid on 'successful participation in the CAP program of interlaboratory testing (Surveys program) required for each analyte whenever an appropriate program is available' and 'It is preferable for the laboratory to have a performance history of one or two quarters prior to the initial inspection'.

On application the laboratory receives the application forms and sectional checklists. The laboratory director distributes the checklist sections to the department heads and asks them to review their department against the checklist to determine whether they meet the criteria for accreditation. Deficiencies should be corrected at this stage as it is the expectation of the Laboratory Accreditation Program that the laboratory will meet the criteria before the on-site inspection. The application questionnaire requires data on personnel, workload, equipment, methodology, proficiency testing, quality control and quality assurance. As described in Chapter 2, a few of the questions are prefixed with LAB (Figure 2.13) and these require completion before the forms are submitted. The application forms plus the partially completed checklists are then returned to the appropriate department in the College of American Pathologists. Preinspection steps in the CPA(UK)Ltd system are similar and have been described briefly at the end of Chapter 3.

THE INSPECTION

The CAP-LAP inspection process begins with the appointment of a team leader who is sent a package of material required for the inspection. This includes a copy of the 'Standards for Laboratory Accreditation', the completed application form of the laboratory to be inspected, partially completed checklists and a summary of the CAP Proficiency programs to which the laboratory subscribes. If it is a re-inspection, then details of the previous visit are included. From this information the team leader has to estimate the time and size of team required for the inspection visit. If the team leader determines that more than one inspector is required then the team leader selects a team which is appropriate to the laboratory to be inspected. Members of the team can be supervisory technologists, clinical scientists, managers, computer specialists, and residents in pathology. Team members do not have to be regular inspectors with the program but they must be aware of the inspection process and knowledgeable in the areas assigned to them for inspection.

CAP-LAP place stress on reviewing the Qualifications of the Director of the laboratory and say that the requirements of Standard I (see Figures 5.5 and 5.6) 'may be more stringent than those established by state and federal governments. This voluntary standard, however, is designed to reflect the optimal rather than the minimal'. Within two weeks of the team leader receiving the information they contact the director and arrange a mutually convenient date for the inspection visit, this is then confirmed in writing. In the CAP-LAP system laboratories who do not submit materials for a reinspection before expiry of their accreditation (within two years of their original accreditation date) are dropped from the program and are required to reapply. There is also an important comment regarding inspection delays, which says 'It is not uncommon for laboratory directors to request delays in inspection due to things such as computer installations, changes in key personnel and mergers. The policy of the Commission on Laboratory Accreditation is that laboratories performing patient testing should be prepared for inspection at any time'.

In CPA(UK)Ltd two inspectors are assigned to each discipline and, if more than one discipline is being inspected, an experienced inspector will act as team leader. Thus if St Elsewhere's Pathology Laboratory were to be inspected, a team of eight inspectors would be required. Of the two inspectors, one is either a pathologist or a clinical scientist of equivalent status and the other from a technical background.

CPA(UK)Ltd's inspection visits are carefully planned in advance and as with CAP-LAP, the receipt of a completed application form is regarded as an indication that the laboratory is ready for inspection. The applicant department is given a clear idea of the nature of the visit and the inspectors in their turn are expected to be familiar with the paperwork from the applicant department and to have identified any points of particular concern. Inspectors are looking for substantial compliance with the standards and must not evaluate the applicant laboratory against their own notions but against the written standards and their interpretative notes.

CAP inspections require meetings with the laboratory director, the hospital administrator (in the case of laboratories closely associated with a hospital) representatives of the medical staff and a walk through the laboratory prior to a detailed inspection. At the end of the inspection a summation conference is held with the laboratory director and other senior personnel at which all the findings of the inspection are reviewed. All significant problems must be identified at the summation conference. It is not surprising that this practice is very similar in CPA(UK)Ltd inspections, as the experience of CAP-LAP was given careful consideration by CPA(UK)Ltd when preparing its own approach. Both CAP-LAP and CPA(UK)Ltd inspections conclude with a summation conference. CAP have the excellent discipline of providing the Director of the applicant department with a photocopy of a summation report at the conference and the applicant laboratories have to send any corrective responses to the CAP office within 30 days of the inspection.

Interview with Managers

During the visits of CPA Inspectors it is important to hold an informal and confidential meeting with the institute manager. This should take no more than 20-30 minutes.

There are two main objectives, to extend common courtesy and to solicit an evaluation of pathology services from the institutional administration point of view.

The basic question is: "Have the pathology staff established an effective working relationship with management?" The following questions may be relevant in this respect:

- How are general relations?
- Are senior professional pathology staff co-operative with managers?
- Are relationships with heads of departments cordial?
- Do you think your pathology services are good?
- Do you see any need for organisational change within pathology in your institution?

These points are leaders for discussion only.

It should be explained that the evaluation and report will take some weeks to be completed and that a full report with recommendations will be returned to the applicant department.

Figure 12.6 CPA(UK)Ltd notes for interview with managers

CPA(UK)Ltd has prepared a leaflet to provide advice to the applicant laboratory's parent body concerning inspection visits. Figures 12.6 and 12.7 indicate what sort of issues might arise in the interviews with managers and with users of the service. This part of the inspection is considered to be of great importance, but an experienced inspector would

Meeting with representatives of the user group

The interview should require no more than 30 minutes and should ask the basic question: "Do local pathology departments provide a good service from your point of view?"

The following questions may be relevant in this respect:

- Are services equally good in all disciplines of pathology or do any stand out as inferior?
- Are clear written instructions available for laboratory users giving advice on what specimens to send, how to send them, what precautions to take, and how much notice is needed?
- Are full and adequate on-call services available in haematology, chemistry and microbiology 24 hours a day, 365 days a year?
- Are there any out-of-hours services in histopathology?
- Is clinical advice available from consultant pathologists (or top grade biochemists) 24 hours a day, 365 days a year?
- Are all such consultants helpful and available?
- Do reports reach their destinations in good time?
- Where appropriate, do they contain adequate supporting information such as normal ranges or clinical comment about an abnormal result?
  - Do pathologists/clinical scientists attend staff rounds?
  - Do pathologists/clinical scientists attend local audit meetings?
  - Are non-clinical laboratory staff helpful and knowledgeable?

It must be stressed that the inspectors are interested in the general quality of the service provided by the laboratory, rather than individual anecdotes, unless such mishaps illustrate a general underlying problem.

Figure 12.7 CPA(UK)Ltd notes for interview with users

know to verify any information given to him at such meetings with commentary from the applicant laboratory. Similarly, when an inspector is looking at a particular aspect of laboratory activity, such as training of staff, it is good practice not only to ask the Head of Department or Director what facilities are available for training staff, but to corroborate that information by interviewing appropriate members of staff to see how the training opportunities are perceived by staff.

POSTINSPECTION

In CAP-LAP, following the on-site inspection, the inspector returns the documentation to the CAP office including the inspector summation report. From this material the staff draft a computerised deficiency commentary which is then provided to the inspection team. Laboratories who do not submit information regarding corrective action within thirty days of the inspection will receive certified letters allowing an additional fifteen days, but continued non-response or incomplete response will result in the recommendation for the denial of accreditation. The Regional Commissioner receives a report which indicates whether the responses to the deficiencies are acceptable and adequate. The commissioner notifies the laboratory that accreditation or a validation inspection is recommended.

The laboratory may challenge the validity of a given deficiency but has to provide documentation to support the challenge. If there is substantial evidence that the deficiency was not valid, the commissioner can elect to have the item removed from the laboratory's record. If, however, a laboratory is cited for more than a certain number of deficiencies, the laboratory is flagged for immediate review by the Regional Commissioner. Possible action can include direct communication with the laboratory director to obtain additional information, a focused reinspection, and in extreme cases a denial of accreditation.

Accreditation is valid for two years from the date of the first inspection, and expires every two years on that anniversary date. Between inspections, that is half way between the two year accreditation period, each laboratory will receive checklists with which to perform a mandatory mid-cycle self-evaluation. These checklists are not returned to the CAP office, but retained by the laboratory along with documentation of corrective action. At the time of the next on-site inspection, these materials are reviewed by the inspector. Many laboratories use the self-evaluation as an educational process, both for staff and pathology residents.

In CPA a similar process takes place. The inspectors compile the report on a discipline basis and they are returned to the central office who then send it to the appropriate specialist advisory committee. These specialist advisory committees have the responsibility of reviewing the inspectors report and advising CPA on whether the laboratory shall be given conditional or full accreditation. In rare instances of serious omissions, the laboratory will be denied accreditation. During the opening phases of CPA's work there has also been what is known as provisional accreditation. This is granted upon receipt of an application form with satisfactory responses to the standards. The granting of provisional accreditation makes it possible to distinguish laboratories that have applied and are awaiting inspection from those who have not made any attempt to progress towards accreditation. The recommendation of the specialist advisory committee is taken to the board for ratification.

In a similar way to the CAP-LAP system, there is an annual registration form to be completed, upon which the laboratory must register all significant changes. These are then studied by central staff and any significant changes in staff, facilities or repertoire discussed with the appropriate specialist advisory committee. This information could result in a limited re-inspection, or an enquiry for further information, until CPA(UK)Ltd is satisfied that the changes indicated in the annual registration form do not significantly alter the accreditation status of that laboratory. At the present time CPA(UK)Ltd is working on a four year cycle of inspection.

MONITORING OF THE INSPECTION PROCESS
In both of the pathology systems there are mechanisms whereby the laboratory that is being inspected can send information regarding the performance of the inspectors to the head office, and this is a way of monitoring the performance of the inspection team.

ISSUES FOR THE ACCREDITATION PROCESS
The whole process of accreditation by peer review involves the provision of inspection staff free of charge, and only travelling expenses and accommodation are refunded. A large number of recognised inspectors or team leaders are required to maintain programmes of this scale, and this will in turn affect the cost of the operation and the frequency with which inspections can be carried out.

The inspector must be thoroughly prepared before his visit. The documentation will often give ideas as to the areas which will require closer scrutiny, and it is helpful if the inspector has some knowledge of the type of equipment being used in the laboratory. If there is more than one inspector looking at a particular department, then there must be a clear division of responsibilities, and a way of the inspectors meshing together again to produce their final report. The inspection process in pathology orientated systems is a peer review process and the discussion is a discussion between equals. It is important to praise good points and innovations in a laboratory to create an atmosphere within which there is no blame attached to some problems, and discussions must be generated by prompting rather than interrogation.

INSPECTORS

SELECTION AND TRAINING
In CAP-LAP, Regional commissioners identify and assign inspection team leaders to the laboratories in their geographical regions. Team leaders must meet defined criteria before being assigned to inspect laboratories, they must be qualified pathologists who are Fellows of the College of American Pathologists and be associated with a CAP accredited laboratory. They must have completed a training programme which provides specific

information about the checklists, the accreditation process and interpretation of the standards. The training programme takes the form of a workshop or seminar and additionally inspectors may be trained on-the-job by a trained inspector. From 1995 monthly seminars have been arranged in major cities across the country in order to give training to non-pathologist inspection team members.

In CPA(UK)Ltd inspectors must be recognised as senior members of their profession and nominations are put forward from professional organisations, these are vetted by the specialist sub committees (see Figure 11.15) before being recommended to the Board for acceptance. Each inspector attends a one day training course which consists of informal presentations followed by group work which might include studying an application form which simulates many of the problems which have been encountered in practice. Inspectors are reimbursed expenses associated with site visits and are expected to make a minimum of two visits per year and attend update sessions which are held in regional centres. Inspectors are selected to be a 'peer' in terms of professional status, size of hospital or laboratory and type of practice and, additionally, should come from a separate region from the applicant laboratory. As the CPA(UK)Ltd scheme matures inspectors are increasingly drawn from accredited laboratories.

INSPECTORS SKILLS

Inspectors should be selected for their knowledge and experience and have good interpersonal skills. Being invited to visit and review performance in a colleague's laboratory is a privilege and the highest standards of personal conduct and confidentiality are required. Inspectors must regard themselves as ambassadors for the particular accreditation system and the way in which they conduct themselves reflects not only on them, but on the organisation for whom they are working.

On the inspection visit first contacts are important and proper introductions should be made and staff should be put at their ease. As there will be a large amount of material to cover, it is important to make it clear to the applicant laboratory staff that things will have to move forward at a steady pace. Information given should be regarded as confidential and inspectors must be totally impartial in the way in which they gather information and comment on it. They should avoid the temptation to impose their own views on the situation and be consistent and objective in the way they work. It is important to try to meet with as many staff as possible because a great deal of effort goes into preparing for accreditation and the staff will regard the inspectors visit as the culmination of that effort. Reports required by the organisation must be sent back promptly to the head office for processing, as failure to do this reflects badly on the whole organisation.

Inspectors must prepare themselves thoroughly for an inspection visit. The content of the application form will sometimes give an early indicator of the strengths and weaknesses of the laboratory. The inspector must be a good listener, must seek to understand the historical background to the current situation, be able to pick up the nuances of concerns and problems, identify which problems are real issues, and avoid being put in a situation where they are manipulated to produce a report on a certain area which the applicant department would like to see. If the inspector is part of a team the work can be allocated according to individual skills. In CAP-LAP and CPA(UK)Ltd inspection is a peer review process and the relationship is between equals, innovations should be praised and when deficiencies are identified they should be discussed with sensitivity and an understanding of the local situation. Finally, an experienced inspector is an educator and should be offering suggestions which might solve problems, by promoting consideration of alternative views, and reflection upon issues. This educational process is an extremely important part of the accreditation process. Being an inspector is also an opportunity to learn!

THE ROAD AHEAD

During the preparation of this book the author has had the opportunity to examine a large amount of material from different quality and accreditation systems and has also had the opportunity to talk to people who have practical experience of the different systems. It is apparent that each system has things of value to offer, but that access is limited by language that is sometimes unfamiliar to the world of clinical pathology.

The importance of ISO 9001 is that it introduces the concept of a quality system which can provide the basis of total quality management. OECD-GLP and other GLP systems bring with them the concept of the formulation of a study plan and the necessity to audit progress in the audit plan and to record data in such a way that assures its integrity and traceability. EN 45001 emphasises a different aspect of traceability in its emphasis on calibration and the accuracy and validity of measurements.

CAP-LAP and CPA(UK), whilst still having things to learn from the other quality and accreditation systems, indicate with their emphasis on the role of the Director of Pathology or head of the discipline and on the pre and post analytic aspects of the process together with participation in proficiency schemes, the breadth of approach required in laboratory medicine. The example of the CAP-LAP scheme is that of an organisation that has accumulated a great amount of practical experience, and as a result has produced a series of checklists which are not only of value in the accreditation process, but also as a way of establishing both vertical and horizontal quality audits in the laboratory. For those who fear over-regulation some peace of mind should accrue from the fact that CAP-LAP as a deemed authority under CLIA'88 is still able to conduct its work in a highly professional and educational manner. It is understood that CAP-LAP will be revising its primary standards in the near future and it will be of great interest to see whether some of the terminology is clarified particularly to fit with international definitions in quality management.

CPA (UK) Ltd. is an organisation that has initially based its standards on the excellent work that has been undertaken in hospital accreditation systems in the United States, Canada, and Australia and by the Kings Fund, London. In the next few years it will undoubtedly have to review its standards in relation to developments which will take place in Europe. The creation of an explicit requirement for a quality manual, and for the appointment of a quality officer in the CAP-LAP and CPA(UK)Ltd systems would firstly provide the opportunity to create a logical structure for the procedures used throughout a laboratory, and the basis of a quality system, secondly ensure the implementation and maintenance of quality systems, and thirdly come closer to the requirements of the internationally recognised quality and accreditation systems.

At present there appears to be at least five groups working in an international or regional context on documents of concern to clinical pathology laboratories. The ISO/IEC Guide 43-1984 (E) which covered guidance on the development and operation of laboratory proficiency testing, with limited emphasis on the use of the outcomes of proficiency testing by accreditation bodies, is also undergoing revision by an ad hoc ISO/CASCO group. The revised guide (voting draft, March 1996) is now intended to provide guidance in three areas:

(1) To distinguish between the use of interlaboratory tests for proficiency testing and for other purposes

(2) To provide guidance on the development and operation of interlaboratory tests for use in proficiency testing schemes

(3) To provide guidance on the selection and use of proficiency testing schemes by laboratory accreditation bodies.

As discussed in Chapter 11 some laboratory accreditation bodies operate their own proficiency schemes but others use proficiency testing schemes or other forms of interlaboratory tests run by other bodies. The purpose of section 2 is to provide harmonised principles for the selection of suitable interlaboratory test programs for use as proficiency testing programmes by accreditation agencies.

With regard to systems for laboratories, four separate groups have been identified by the author. In 1994 WELAC now EAL (see Figure 12.1) formed a joint working party with the European Confederation of Laboratory Medicine (ECLM) and have produced a draft document 'Comments to facilitate its (ISO/IEC Guide 25) use in a clinical laboratory environment'. The group state that the document 'is intended to provide guidance for assessors and laboratories on the specific interpretation of ISO/IEC Guide 25 (*'General requirements for the competence of calibration and testing laboratories'*) in the field of laboratory medicine. The aim is that it should be generally applicable for quality management in every field of laboratory medicine whenever accreditation according to ISO/IEC Guide 25 applies'. In addition to this activity the ISO/IEC Guide 25 is itself undergoing revision by Work Group 10 of the ISO committee for conformity assessment (CASCO).

Secondly, another group, ISO TC 212 Work Group 1 Task group 3, is preparing an intended international document on Quality assurance in clinical laboratory proficiency and accreditation.

The document intends to address,

- internal quality control procedures
- external quality assurance, including proficiency testing and quality assessment
- requirements for accreditation
- nonanalytical performance indicators, including turnaround time, practicability and utilisation management

In the draft of the 20th April 1996 some of the broader issues in laboratory medicine are being discussed.

A third group is operating under the aegis of the International Union of Pure and Applied Chemistry (IUPAC). In the Clinical Chemistry section, the Commission on components of quality systems in the clinical laboratory has produced a commentary on ISO 9004-5 (Quality management and quality system elements Part 5: Guidelines for quality plans) entitled 'Quality Management and Quality System Elements in the Clinical Laboratory-Guideline for Quality plans'. A quality plan is defined in ISO 8402;1994 as a document setting out the specific quality practices, resources and sequences of activities relevant to a particular product, project or contract. In the introduction to the commentary it draws attention to the OECD-GLP definition of Standard Operating Procedures as 'written procedures which describe how to perform certain routine laboratory tests or activities normally not specified in detail in study plans or test guidelines' and claims that this shows the relationship between quality plans and standard operating procedures. However, that implies that a study plan is equivalent to a quality plan. The OECD-GLP definition of a study plan is 'a document which defines the entire scope of the study'; with this definition only in a very limited sense would a study plan be the same as a quality plan.

Finally, the Working Group on Harmonisation of Quality Systems and Accreditation of the European Communities Confederation of Clinical Chemistry (EC4) has published 'Essential Criteria for Quality Systems of Clinical Biochemistry Laboratories in the EU'. Although the title indicates an apparent limitation of this document to clinical chemistry, it has been written in such a way that it could be used for all disciplines in pathology. The document is reproduced in Appendix 5 and inspection will show that in addition to covering all the items required in a quality/accreditation system for laboratory medicine, it is cross referenced to EN 45001:1989, ISO 9000 series standards and to the third draft of the revised ISO/IEC Guide 25.

As mentioned in Chapter 11 within the European Community precedents already exist for the harmonisation of laws, regulations and administrative provisions relating to the application of the principles of Good Laboratory Practice and to the inspection and verification of Good Laboratory Practice. The adoption of a similar Directive giving the essential criteria for quality and accreditation systems for clinical pathology laboratories, together with a requirement for harmonisation of laws, regulations and administrative provisions in respect of the conduct of clinical pathology, would lead to member states examining their current provision. Once harmonisation is achieved, then the principle of subsidiarity (allowing decisions to be made at the lowest practicable level) would allow member states within such a framework to make the appropriate arrangements for verification of compliance with the essential criteria. This could be done by regulation or by license or by giving deemed status to an appropriate body such as CPA(UK)Ltd.

The 'Road Ahead' looks set to have many road works and diversions which will impede progress, but as Bill Gates says at the end of his book concerning the information highway, 'The network will draw us together, if that's what we choose, or let us scatter ourselves into a million mediated communities'. The choice is ours!

FURTHER READING

EN 45002:1989, General criteria for the assessment of testing laboratories.

EN 45003:1989, General criteria for laboratory accreditation bodies.

EN 45012:1989, General criteria for certification bodies operating quality system certification.

Good Laboratory Practice: The United Kingdom compliance programme 1989, Department of Health.

Introducing NAMAS M1 1989, NAMAS/DTI (see Appendix 1 for address).

Laboratory Accreditation Manual, Commission on Laboratory Accreditation; ed T E Campbell, 1994, College of American Pathologists.

Strategic Review of Pathology Services 1995, NHS Executive, HMSO London.

UKAS - Memorandum of understanding, UKAS Update Edition 1, October 1996. United Kingdom Accreditation Service.

United Kingdom Accreditation Service Introductory leaflet 1995.

Appendix 1

Useful addresses

The following are addresses of some of the main sources of information in this book.

Advisory,Conciliation and Arbitration Service,
(ACAS)
Head Office,
27 Wilton Street,
London SW1X 7AZ
United Kingdom

Association of Clinical Biochemists,
2 Carlton House Terrace,
London SW2Y 5AF
United Kingdom

British Standards Institution,
389 Chiswick High Road,
London W4 4AL
United Kingdom

College of American Pathologists,
325 Waukegan Road,
Northfield, Illinois 60093-2750,
USA

European Committee for Standardization (CEN)
Rue de Stassart, 36,
B-1050 Bruxelles,
Belgium

The Industrial Society,
Robert Hyde House,
48 Bryanston Square,
London W1H 7LN

Medical Devices Agency, (Department of Health),
Hannibal House,
Elephant and Castle,
London SE1 6TQ
United Kingdom

American Association of Clinical Chemistry Inc.,
(CAP)
2101 L St., Suite 202,
Washington, DC 20037-1526
USA

Audit Commission,
1 Vincent Square,
London SW1P 2PN
United Kingdom

Clinical Pathology Accreditation (UK) Ltd.,
Pathology Block,
The Childrenís Hospital,
Western Bank,
Sheffield S10 2TH
United Kingdom

Commission on Office Laboratory Accreditation,
(COLA)
1707 Main Street/Suite 406,
Longmont, CO 80501,
USA

Health and Safety Executive Books,
P.O. Box 1999, Sudbury,
Suffolk CO10 6PS
United Kingdom

International Laboratory Accreditation
Conference
Secretariat ILAC 96
c/o NKO/STERIN/STERLAB
P O Box 29152,
3001 GD Rotterdam,
The Netherlands

National Pathology Accreditation Advisory
Council,
Secretary NPAAC, P O Box 658,
Woden ACT 2606
Australia

NCCLS
940 West Valley Road,
Suite 1400,
Wayne, PA 19087-1878,
USA

Organisation for Economic Co-operation and
Development (OECD),
2 Rue Andre Pascal,
75775 Paris Cedex 16,
France

Office for Official Publications of the European
Communities,
2 rue Mercier,
L-2985, Luxembourg

The Royal College of Pathologists,
2 Carlton House Terrace,
London SW1Y 5AF
United Kingdom

Appendix 2

Comparison of paragraphs in international guides and standards

This table below is modified from:- CITAC Guide 1 , International Guide to Quality in Analytical Chemistry An Aid to Accreditation, ISBN 0 948926 09 0, December 1995.

for further information contact Mr David Holcombe, Drafting Secretary of the CITAC Working Group, Laboratory of the Government Chemist, Queens road, Teddington, Middlesex TW11 0LY United Kingdom. (CITAC Co-operation on International Traceability in Analytical Chemistry).

	ISO/IEC Guide 25	ISO 9001:1994	OECD-GLP
Management and organisation	4	4.1	1
Quality system			
• Audit and review	5.2-5.6	4.1, 4.17	2.2, 9.2
• Quality Manager	5.1	4.1	1.1, 2
• Quality Manual	5.2	4.2	2.1
Staff	6	4.18	1.1, 1.3
Environment	7	4.11h, 4.11j	3.1-3.4
Equipment	8	4.11	4.1
Calibration and traceability	9	4.11b, c, e-g	4.1, 7.2
Test methods	10	4.7-4.11	2.2, 4.1, 6.1, 6.2, 7, 8
Sample handling	11	4.8, 4.10, 4.15,	6.1
Records	12	4..5, 4.16	3.4, 9, 10
Reports	13	4.10.4, 4.16	3.4, 9, 10
Subcontracting	14	4.6.2	
Support services	15	4.6, 4.7	
Complaints	16	4.13, 4.14	

Appendix 3

The Retention and Storage of Pathological Records and Archives

REPORT OF THE WORKING PARTY OF THE ROYAL COLLEGE OF PATHOLOGISTS

Published by the Royal College of Pathologists Marks and Spencer Publications Unit (February 1995). Copies of the Report available from The Royal College of Pathologists, 2 Carlton House Terrace, London SW1Y 5AF., ISBN 0 9518574 3 6.

TERMS OF REFERENCE

The Working Party was appointed by the Council of the Royal College of Pathologists with the following terms of reference:

> *"To make recommendations on minimum retention times for pathology records, tissues, and semi-permanent or permanent pathological preparations, including those required for operational use, for education, teaching, training and general scholarship, for research per se, for historical purposes and against the possibility of future litigation, audit or allegations of scientific fraud and to report to Council".*

WORKING PARTY

Professor Dame Rosalinde Hurley *Chairman*
Professor Sir Colin Berry
Dr. N.J. Dodd
Mr. I. Dodds-Smith *(McKenna and Co)*
Professor B.I. Duerden
Dr. J.D.S. Kay
Dr. A. McDermott

Observers
Dr. Phyllis Furnell *(Department of Health)*
Dr. Aileen Keel *(Scottish Office)*
Dr. J. Pritchard *(Welsh Office)*

The Report has been prepared on their behalf by Professor Dame Rosalinde Hurley and Dr. Jonathan Kay.

THE WORKING PARTY CONSIDERED THE FOLLOWING DOCUMENTS:

i) Department of Health, Health Circular, HC(80)7: Retention of Personal Health Records *(for possible use in litigation)*. Amending HM(61)73 and HM(65)71.

ii) Department of Health, Health Circular, HC(89)20: *Preservation, Retention and Destruction of Records, Responsibilities of Health Authorities under the Public Records Acts*. Cancels HM(61)73, HN(76)48 and HC(80)7.

iii) Bulletin of the Royal College of Pathologists: (a) June 1977 *Retention of copies of laboratory reports;* (b) September 1985 *Retention of human tissue removed at operation;* (c) June 1986 *Signing reports;* (d) April 1990 *Retention of post mortem material.*

iv) HN(88)3: *Procurement Product Liability.*

v) *Guidelines for the release of laboratory test results, reports and specimens to patients, interested groups and organisations.* Canadian Medical Association Journal 1990; 143 (9):847-848.

vi) General Medical Council News Review, December 1992 *The use of facsimile machines in the transmission of confidential information.*

vii) Guidance of the College of American Pathologists including: *Federal Law Requirements under the Clinical Laboratory Improvement Act and Professional Relations Manual* 9th Edition 1988.

viii) *Guidance for the retention and destruction of health records.* (MEL(1933)152) Scottish Office.

x) *Risk Management in the NHS.* NHSME 1993.

xi) *Correspondence* from the Chief Medical Officer to the President of the Royal College of Physicians, 1993.

xii) *Population Needs and Genetic Services.* An outline Guide (PL/CM093/5) - Services for Genetic Disorders.

xiii) *The Medical Museum and its relevance to modern medicine.* Turk, JL. Journal of the Royal Society of Medicine 1994; 87:40-42.

xiv) General Medical Council: *Professional Conduct and Discipline: Fitness to practise.* paragraph 78, as amended (Annual Report, 1992, p.4).

xv) British Committee for Standards in Haematology

    a) *Guidelines for compatibility testing in Hospital Blood Banks.*

      Clinical and Laboratory Haematology 1987; 9:333-341.

    b) *Guidelines on Hospital Blood Bank documentation and procedures.*

      Clinical and Laboratory Haematology 1990; 12:209-220.

    c) *Guidelines on product liability for the Hospital Blood Bank.*

      Clinical and Laboratory Haematology 1990; 12:329-344.

xvi) *BSCC Recommended Code of practice for Laboratories providing a cytopathology service* 1986. BSCC Secretariat.

xvii) *Retention of Pathology Records:* Documentation, Reports, Specimens and Tissues. A note on essential issues and the legal background by the Chairman. 1994.

The Working Party took account of the Control of Substances Hazardous to Health Regulations 1988 S11988 No. 1657, the Health and Safety at Work Act 1974, the Congenital Disabilities (Civil Liability) Act 1976, the Limitation Act 1975, The Consumer Protection Act 1987, the Access to Health Records Act 1990, Human Tissue Act 1961, Data Protection Act 1984, Health Building Note 15 Guidance on Accommodation for Pathology Services, paragraph 4.91.

Dr. Kenneth Calman, Chief Medical Officer (England) has advised in correspondence that the principles in the Department of Health's guidance on Preservation, Retention and Destruction of Records HC(89)20 apply with equal force both to the preservation of paper records and to the preservation of non-paper records such as pathology material and other biological samples which provides a record of a patient, adding that information which seems likely to provide material for medical research should be scrutinised with a view to permanent preservation, and acknowledging the value to genetic services of retaining informative medical records and biological samples where resources are available for this. The Working Party finds the Chief Medical Officer's guidance particularly helpful and apposite in its general context, and, also, in its admonition that we should look at future research endeavour, especially in the field of preservation of material that may yield information of genetic importance (preservation of samples that may yield DNA for future analysis or otherwise be available for study).

Health Authorities have been asked to review their procedures periodically so that records appropriate for retention beyond the recommended minimum periods should be reached locally and we concur, and commend this to pathologists. There are resource implications for the retention of records and of biological specimens and available resources will have to be taken into account in such reviews.

The Public Records Acts 1958 and 1967 contain the procedure for the preservation of public records and for authorisation of the destruction of those that are no longer required. HC(89)20 enjoins on health authorities the duty to designate an officer to make appropriate arrangements for the selection and permanent preservation of public records and to liaise as necessary with the Public Record Office. Under no circumstance may a record older than 1660 be destroyed and the Local Records Office should be consulted before records more than 60 years old are destroyed. With respect to historical pathological archives this is an important safeguard.

THE SCOPE AND NATURE OF PATHOLOGY RECORDS INCLUDES:

I) CLINICAL AND DIAGNOSTIC RECORDS AND REPORTS

These are hard copy reports or electronic records of the results of pathological investigation(s) sent or made available to the requesting clinicians. With respect to computer generated records, the same criteria that cover conventional records apply, unless they have been converted already to hard copy records and preserved as such. If held only on microfilm, microfiche or original magnetic data files, extra care is needed to prevent corruption or deterioration of data. As equipment becomes obsolete, re-recording may need to be considered. The minimum periods of retention specified for certain categories of patients are embodied in HC(89)20 and HC(80)7, and are summarised in the Appendix. Hard copy reports of pathological investigations for these categories of patients should be incorporated in their individual clinical records and, although there is no obligation to destroy them at all, patient records may not be destroyed until the minimum period for retention has elapsed.

II) LABORATORY RECORDS: REPORTS, DOCUMENTATION, SPECIMENS
include request forms; protocols of procedures, day books; work sheets; batch records; stored specimens such as serum, tissues, blocks, wet preparations; stained slides or other permanent or semi-
permanent preparations; photographic records; museum specimens; the pathological
archive/museum catalogues; bound copies of reports/records; near-patient test data; correspondence; records of telephoned reports; test cards (neonatal screening for phenylketonuria, the
Guthrie test card); cultures, freeze dried or otherwise preserved, or short term; equipment maintenance logs; quality control and quality assurance records; accreditation documents; records of
inspections. Financial records, invoices, stores issues and the like are the subject of separate guidance under HC(89)20 and are not considered further.

Diagnostic records are properly retained in individual patient notes or in electronic form the safe
keeping of which is the responsibility of hospital records departments or recipient general practitioners or private practitioners, once the pathologist has issued the reports. Where pathologists
have reason to doubt the reliability of systems of patient record keeping they should bring this to
the attention of those responsible rather than attempt to rectify it by duplication and local and prolonged laboratory storage of diagnostic records.

There are reasons why individual pathologists or heads of departments may wish to retain documents or materials either in the short term, or permanently. They include:

    i)   further diagnosis, or ongoing clinical management

    ii)   clinical audit

    iii)   teaching and comparative research, including epidemiology

    iv)   analysis of data (such as casemix) for administrative or other purposes

    v)   direct evidence in litigation

    vi)   research data, kept on file

    vii) historical purposes

    viii) good clinical laboratory practice

    x)   review

Need will vary according to the discipline of pathology that is practised. Where specimens or permanent or semi-permanent preparations are kept they must be adequately labelled, indexed and
catalogued, so that the record remains accessible and usable.

The recommendations that follow refer to the **MINIMUM** times of retention that are consonant
with acceptable practice. If any of our recommendations indicate a shorter time for retention than
those required by recognised systems of good laboratory practice, such as NAMAS, we recommend
that the latter be followed by subscribing laboratories. Many pathologists will have good and
cogent reasons for retaining records and materials for much longer periods. Where laboratories or
hospitals are to be closed, we recommend that pathologists discuss with responsible managers the
need to retain and relocate records and materials, so that continuity of essential data storage is
maintained and the records remain accessible at all times. This will necessitate careful organisation.

MINIMUM RETENTION TIMES

(see section entitled 'Long-term (permanent) retention of records' for explanation of the term 'permanently')

A.   DOCUMENTS AND PAPER RECORDS

(see also Sections C and D, blood transfusion laboratories and forensic material)

- **Request forms**

  It is prudent to keep request forms until the authorised report has been received by the requester. As this period of time may vary with local circumstances we do not recommend a minimum retention time but believe that, ordinarily, request forms need not be kept for longer than one month after the final checked report has been despatched. For most laboratories, retention for one week should suffice. Where the request form contains clinical information not readily accessible in the patient's notes, but used in the interpretation of test data (as in screening for alpha fetoprotein) the request should be kept permanently.

- **Day Books and other record of specimens received by a laboratory**

  Two calendar years.

- **Protocols of Standard Operating Procedures**

  Both current and outdated protocols should be dated and kept permanently on file.

- **Worksheets**

  Keep for same length of time as related permanent or semi-permanent specimens or preparations.

- **Laboratory File cards or other working record of test results for named patients**

  Two calendar years.

- **Records of telephoned reports**

  Log on patient's file card or other working records.

- **Reports, copies**

  Six months for operational purposes; permanently for historical or research.

- **Surgical (histological) reports**

  Hard copy lodged in patient's notes. Bound copies of reports kept permanently by the laboratory.

- **Post mortem reports**

  Report should be lodged in patient's record. Bound copies of reports kept permanently.

- **Correspondence on patients**

  Should be lodged in patient's record. Otherwise, keep permanently.

- **Near-patient test data**

  Results should be entered on patient's record; log should be retained for lifetime of instrument.

- **Bound copies of reports/records**

  Permanently.

- **Pathological archive/museum catalogues**

  Permanently.

- **Photographic records**

  Permanently.

- **Batch records**
  Permanently.

- **Internal quality Control Records**
  Permanently.

- **External Quality Assurance Records**
  Two calendar years.

- **Accreditation documents; records of inspections**
  Ten years.

- **Equipment maintenance logs**
  Lifetime of instrument.

- **Records of service inspections, maintenance of instruments**
  Ten years.

- **On-line diagnostic electronic records**
  Six months. Hard copy reports should be made to notes.

- **Neonatal Screening Test Cards**
  Twenty years or longer if no deterioration has occurred. Such cards may be useful as sources of DNA for retrospective analysis and research.

- **Records relevant to production of products (diagnostics) or equipment**
  Comprehensive records relevant to procurement, use, modification and supply: eleven years.

- **Research data**
  see below.

- **Records relating to organ transplantation**
  Records not otherwise kept or issued to patient records that relate to investigations or storage of specimens relevant to organ transplantation or retention of semen or ova should be kept permanently.

B. SPECIMENS AND PREPARATION
(see also Sections C and D, blood transfusion laboratories and forensic material)

- **Plasma/serum/bodily fluids/swabs**
  Forty eight hours after final report has been issued by the laboratory.

- **Wet Tissue**
  Four weeks after final report.

- **Whole blood samples, for full blood count**
  Twenty four hours.

- **Frozen sections (unless further processed)**
  Four weeks after final report.

- **Paraffin blocks; blocks for electron microscopy, DNA analysis**
  Permanently; minimum lifetime of patient. It is important that specimens for DNA analysis be stored for later analysis of mutations in patients with familial cancers. Such samples should be held for five years after the death of the patient.

- **Museum specimens**
  Permanently.

- **Stained slides**

a)	microbiological:	Seven days after final report.
b)	blood films, routine:	Seven days after final report.
c)	cytogenetic preparations:	Two years after final report, if photographic record kept; five years otherwise.
d)	bone marrow smears:	Twenty years minimum; ideally over lifetime of patient.
e)	cytology, including population screening	Ten years minimum, longer if possible, to cover at least one recall visit.
f)	histology:	Ten years; permanently if practicable.
		Unstained (spare) sections and electron microscopy sections kept similarly.

- **Serum**
  That from the first pregnancy booking visit should be kept for one calendar year to provide a base-line for further serological or other tests for infections or other disease during pregnancy and after delivery. Fetal serum (cordocentesis) should be kept permanently. Serum taken after needlestick injury or other hazardous exposure should be kept for a minimum of two years. Other left-over sera or plasma should be stored for as long as practicable to provide an array of material for future research. *(see also Section C)*

- **Human DNA**
  Four weeks after final report for diagnostic specimens; permanently if to be used for research or if specifically needed for family studies in those with genetic disorders. The need for retention of diagnostic specimens should be assessed at the time of issuing the final report. Specimens that were used in a linkage study should be kept for ten years, and research specimens permanently.

- **Microbiological cultures**
  Most positive cultures can be discarded within 24-48 hours of issuing a final authorised report. Specified cultures of clinical importance (blood culture isolates, CSF isolates, enteric pathogens, multiply or methicillin resistant Staph.aureus, 'outbreak' strains, M.tuberculosis, Group A streptococci, and unusual pathogens of clinical significance) should be retained for at least seven days.

- **Freeze dried or other permanently preserved cultures**
  Permanently.

C. DOCUMENTS, PAPER RECORDS, SPECIMENS AND PREPARATIONS: SPECIFIC ADVICE FOR TRANSFUSION LABORATORIES

Minimum requirements for retention times may differ from those detailed in Sections A and B; in all instances the longer period is recommended.

- **Request forms for grouping, antibody screening and cross-matching**
  One month.

- **Work sheets**
  Eleven years.

- **Results of grouping and antibody screening**
  Permanently.

- **Blood Bank Register**
  Eleven years.

- **Refrigeration Charts**
  Eleven years.

- **Freezer Charts**
  Eleven years.

- **Clotted blood for grouping, antibody screening and saving and/or cross-matching**
  One week at 4°C.

- **Serum from requests for grouping, antibody screening and saving**
  One week, optimally at -30°C or colder.

- **Serum for cross-matching**
  No minimum time is recommended. Storage should optimally be at -30°C or colder. May be stored for up to one month, and occasionally longer, prior to a planned procedure, provided no blood components are given during this time and that the patient has not been transfused or pregnant in the preceding four months.

- **Serum following a cross-match or transfusion**
  One week. Storage should optimally be at -30°C or colder. This serum may only be used for the investigation of transfusion reactions and not for further cross-matching.

D. FORENSIC MATERIAL

Autopsy reports, specimens, archive material and other whether the deceased has been the subject of a Coroner's or Fiscal autopsy

HM Coroners or Procurators Fiscal have absolute dominion over autopsy reports. They are confidential to them and may not be released without their consent to any third party. We believe that it is good practice to lodge copies of forensic autopsy reports in the deceased's notes but the consent of the Coroner or Procurator Fiscal should be obtained. Such consent may be refused. In Scotland, we know that the Procurator's Fiscal permit the full text of the autopsy report to be issued to the nominated regional paediatrician in cases of Sudden Infant Death Syndrome; reports on maternal deaths are issued to appropriate National Enquiry Committees. We commend these practices.

Tissues which have a bearing upon the investigation of the cause of death must be retained under the 1984 Coroners' rules (Rule 9) until the completion of the inquest in England. In deaths subject to criminal enquiry, relevant material must be retained until both Coroner's interest has expired and other interests such as those of the Crown Prosecution Service have been fulfilled, these varying from case to case.

TEACHING RECORDS

Selected photographs, preserved cultures, mounted specimens and stained slides, with the blocks pertaining in the case of surgical pathology are an invaluable resource and should be lodged, adequately indexed, described and catalogued, in permanent collections either in the laboratory of first instance or in local, central or national archives.

RESEARCH DATA AND RECORDS

Confidential named patient data (documentation) collected in the course of investigation and held separately from patients' records should be destroyed or anonymised six months after the research has been completed, the data analysed, and final publication of findings has been made. Working records and other research data should be retained permanently to rebut allegations of scientific fraud if such are made. Records of clinical trial data must be kept for fifteen years. The provisions of the Data Protection Act (1984) must be observed for these as for other pathological records.

CONFIDENTIALITY OF RECORDS

The General Medical Council instructs that "doctors carry a prime responsibility for the protection of information given to them by patients or obtained in confidence about patients. They must therefore take steps to ensure, as far as lies in their control, that the records, manual or computerised, which they keep, to which they have access, or which they transmit are protected by effective security systems with adequate procedures to prevent improper disclosure". Confidential information on patients may be transmitted by fax or from one computer to another. It is important to ensure that the information is sent to the correct location and that only the intended recipient will be able to access it. Both sender and recipient must establish arrangements to allow this. The primary responsibility lies with the sender and a key step is to establish that the receiving fax transreceiver is in a 'safe haven'.

In the case of non-paper records the pathologist has a duty to ensure that specimens are kept not only confidentially but safely and securely so as to guard against accidental or non-accidental mishap. Some items (e.g. cultures of viable organisms) may need to be stored in locked containers. The provisions of the COSHH regulations and of Health and Safety at Work legislation must be observed.

LONG TERM (PERMANENT) RETENTION OF RECORDS

Retention of records beyond thirty years, other than in the case of recognised historical archives already kept in approved places of deposit, (which may include the premises of medical institutions), requires an application to the Lord Chancellor through the Keeper of Public Records if there is need for them to be retained by a Health Authority rather than transferred to a place of deposit or destroyed.

Pathologists should therefore be prepared to cause records to be destroyed after thirty years unless they wish to state a case for their further retention, or unless the records under their immediate care are already secured in an approved place of deposit.

Property in pathological materials and records, as in other Health Service (NHS) records and items, vests ultimately in the Secretary of State for Health. The long term retention of documentary material is subject to the guidance of the Keeper of Public Records. Usage of pathological material, held by pathologists, for research, teaching or scholarship and the ethical considerations pertaining, if any, are not matters that the present Working Party can or is willing to address in this report other than to advise that consideration be given to long term retention of material of potential value in genetic or other research. Property in records, reports and materials relating to procedures within the jurisdiction of an appointed and legally competent authority (Coroner, Procurator Fiscal) does not vest in the same way. Pathologists will wish to bear this distinction in mind.

APPENDIX

MINIMUM RETENTION PERIODS: PERSONAL HEALTH RECORDS: DEPARTMENT OF HEALTH GUIDANCE

i) **Obstetric records:** twenty five years.

ii) **Records relating to children and young people (including paediatric, vaccination and community child health service records):** until the patient's 25th birthday if an entry was made when the young person was 17, that is, before the 18th birthday.

iii) **Records relating to mentally disordered persons within the meaning of the Mental health Act 1959:** twenty years from the date at which, in the opinion of the doctor concerned, the disorder has ceased or diminished to the point where no further care or treatment is considered necessary.

Except that such records need only be retained for a minimum of seventy eight years after the death of a patient (or, in the case of obstetric records, death of the child - but not of the mother).

iv) **All other personal health records:** eight years after the conclusion of treatment. After the appropriate minimum period has expired the need to retain them further for local use should be carefully and if necessary periodically, reviewed. Because of the sensitivity and confidential nature of such records and the need to ensure that decisions on retention balance the interests of professional staff, including any research in which they are or may be engaged, and the resources available for storage, some health authorities have established committees to oversee the procedures for the retention and destruction of these records. Others may wish to consider if it would be helpful to do so.

As records could be required in litigation virtually without limit of time, the Department recognises that some records may be destroyed that might otherwise subsequently have been required for litigation. The Department's view however, is that the cost of indefinite retention of records should greatly exceed the liabilities likely to be incurred in the occasional case where defence and action for damages is handicapped by the absence of records. If a hospital doctor involved in litigation claims that prior disposal of relevant medical records has prejudiced the outcome, this should be considered by the health authority along with all other factors when the appointment of any liability as between the doctor and health authority is being contemplated.

Acknowledgement

The Working Party wishes to record its indebtedness to Ian Dodds-Smith of McKenna and Company, Solicitors, who gave freely of his time and expertise in this matter.

Appendix 4

Guidelines for the Approval of External Quality Assessment Schemes

JOINT WORKING GROUP ON QUALITY ASSURANCE (UK)
(Secretary, c/o Diagnostic Services Ltd, Mast House, Darby Road ,Liverpool L20 1EA)

External Quality Assessment (EQA) Schemes are an essential component of measures to ensure acceptable standards of laboratory performance. They allow for objective assessment of laboratory performance and have an important educational role. Approved schemes must comply with the following criteria.

1. A scheme must have input from appropriate professional advisors (nominated by or accepted by the Joint Working Group and the appropriate Advisory Panel) to ensure acceptable standards of scheme design, organisation and management (ie a Steering Committee).

2. A scheme must regularly submit summarised results and reports to the appropriate National Quality Assurance Advisory Panel with whom it must agree appropriate standards of performance and participation and methods for the monitoring of both. The arrangements must also include the provision of advice and assistance to participants when requested or necessary.

3. A scheme must provide regular distributions at acceptable intervals of material designed to test an appropriate range of diagnostic procedures and/or analyses in the field in which it operates.

4. The material distributed in a scheme should be of as consistent a matrix as possible and resemble as closely as is practicable the relevant clinical material. It must also conform with all relevant UK safety standards and provisions.

5. Data must be presented to participants in a timely and easily understood manner.

6. A scheme must offer participants regular opportunities to comment on the scheme to the organisers and to contribute to scheme development.

7. Participants must be identified by a code, which is confidential between the Scheme Organisers, the particpant and in certain circumstances the Panel Chairman. Where appropriate the code should be common to other relevant recognised schemes.

8. The continuing approval of a scheme will be subject to periodic scrutiny to ensure continuing compliance with the above criteria.

NB: Schemes which are not independent of manufacturing and marketing interests in equipment, reagents or kits in the participating field may be approved provided that they meet the above requirements. When a scheme is run by an organisation with commerical interests (such as in equipment or reagents) in the field in which other schemes operate, that organisation must derive no deliberate advantage in its other commercial activities from the running of the scheme. Such a separation of interests must be clearly demonstrable and will be under a constant surveillance.

Appendix 5

Essential Criteria for Quality Systems of Clinical Biochemistry Laboratories in the EU

EUROPEAN COMMUNITIES CONFEDERATION OF CLINICAL CHEMISTRY (EC4)

Prepared by the Working Group on Harmonisation of Quality Systems and Accreditation
May 1996 © EC4

Dr. R.T.P. Jansen (NVKC, Netherlands), Chairman

Prof.dr. V. Blaton (BVKC, Belgium)   Dr. J.M. Queraltó (SEBCPM, Spain)

Dr. D. Burnett (ACB, United Kingdom)   Dr. S. Zérah (SFBC, France)

Dr. W. Huisman (NVKC, Netherlands)   Dr. B. Allman (EDMA), observer

---

SECTION

0.   Introduction and scope

1.   General information

2.   Quality policy and strategy

3.   Organization and management

4.   Personnel

5.   Premises and environment

6.   Equipment, materials and reagents

7.   Pre-analytical phase

8.   Analytical phase

9.   Post-analytical phase

10.   Evaluation of the quality system

0. Introduction and scope

There is increasing awareness in medical laboratories for the need of total quality management. After a long history of the use of internal quality control and external quality assessment schemes, there is now the requirement for control of the complete laboratory process. An important tool to achieve such control is a total quality management system. Medical laboratories are in need of international criteria for such quality systems.

There exist International Standards for certification (ISO 9001) and for accreditation (EN 45001 and ISO Guide 25). However these standards are either very general (ISO 9001), or are developed for testing and calibration laboratories (EN 45001, ISO Guide 25), and therefore do not address specific aspects of the work of medical laboratories. The scope of medical and clinical laboratories is different from these laboratories and needs additional criteria.

The Working Group on Harmonisation of Quality and Accreditation Systems of The European Communities Confederation of Clinical Chemistry (EC4) has prepared the present document in order to clarify the specific needs. This document provides guidelines for implementation of total quality systems in clinical biochemistry laboratories. Although written for clinical biochemistry laboratories it is easily applicable for multidisciplinary and other types of medical laboratories. The quality systems of medical laboratories should reflect the special tasks of such laboratories. Therefore the emphasis of the document is not only on analytical and observational aspects, but also on the pre-analytical and post-analytical phases, on consultation and on efficacy and efficiency of requested investigations.

Where possible, reference is given to EN 45001, ISO Guide 25 (Draft 3) and ISO 9001 standards. Several criteria are not addressed in these standards. In particular additional to the ISO Guide 25 and the EN 45001 standards are criteria in Sections 7 and 9 of this document concerning the pre- and post-analytical phases, but also criteria in other sections concerning patient preparation, clinical advice, efficacy and teaching, are additional.

Some requirements of the EN 45001 standard and ISO Guide 25 seem less relevant for medical laboratories. Requirements regarding calibration are formulated differently in the present document. This also pertains to the reference methods and materials requirements, which in many cases are not available for medical laboratory tests, particularly the observational. The use of subcontractors for specialized or infrequently requested assays is daily practice for medical laboratories, contrary to requirements for testing laboratories.

A medical laboratory that has implemented a quality system according to the criteria described in the present document, fulfils ISO 9001, EN 45001 and ISO Guide 25 standards that are relevant to medical laboratories, and is prepared for accreditation or certification by all relevant schemes. Particularly schemes originating, though independently operating, from the professions, like the Belgian system, CCKLtest in the Netherlands, CPA in the United Kingdom, the French GBEA system, are suited for such accreditation. Guidelines published by these organisations are in agreement with the present international document and the Handbooks and Model Quality Manuals based on the guidelines and issued in these countries are of use for laboratories wishing to implement a quality system based on the present document.

1. General information

1.1 Introduction

1.2 Definitions and abbreviations

1.3 Legal identity

1.4 Clinical advisory service based on analytical facilities

1.5 Research and development

1.6 Teaching

1.7 Subcontractors

1.1 INTRODUCTION
- There should be a description of the scope of the quality system, the use of the quality manual and the relationship to the quality system of the parent organization if applicable. (addressed in ISO 9001 1)

1.2 DEFINITIONS AND ABBREVIATIONS
- Used terms should be defined. (addressed in EN 45001 2; ISO Guide 25 3; ISO 9001 3)

- Used abbreviations should be explained. (addressed in EN 45001 2; ISO Guide 25 3; ISO 9001 3)

1.3 LEGAL IDENTITY
- The legal identity (type, name, address) of the laboratory should be stated. (addressed in EN 45001 3; ISO Guide 25 4.1; ISO 9001 4.1)

- Name and title of the director of the laboratory should be stated. (addressed in ISO Guide 25 4.2)

- The position of the laboratory within the parent organization should be clarified, e.g. in an organizational diagram.

1.4 CLINICAL ADVISORY SERVICE BASED ON ANALYTICAL FACILITIES
- There should be a list of activities of the laboratory with respect to the covered fields and clinical advice.

- There should be a list of the general methodologies and techniques used.

- A list should be available of the repertoire in regular and out of hours service.

- The types of requesting physicians and if applicable other service users should be stated.

1.5 RESEARCH AND DEVELOPMENT
- The laboratory is recommended to take part regularly in projects of research concerning development or evaluation of new methods and methodologies.

- Larger laboratories should be involved in research.

- If applicable the hospital laboratory should give support to clinical research.

- The laboratory should give analytical and consulting support to clinical trials.

1.6 TEACHING
- The laboratory should take part in teaching of medical students, nurses, technologists and trainees if applicable.

1.7 SUBCONTRACTORS
- There should be a list of activities performed by subcontractors.
  (addressed in EN 45001 5.4.7; ISO Guide 25 14.2)

- Subcontractors should be known, recognized or accredited institutes or laboratories.
  (addressed in EN 45001 5.4.7; ISO Guide 25 14.1)

2. Quality policy and strategy

2.1 Quality policy of the parent organization

2.2 Quality policy of the laboratory

2.3 Quality strategy of the laboratory

2.4 Confidentiality

2.5 Improper influence

2.1 QUALITY POLICY OF THE PARENT ORGANIZATION
- There should be a list of references to quality documents of the parent organization, if applicable.

2.2 QUALITY POLICY OF THE LABORATORY
- The general policy of the laboratory with regard to quality issues should include services, health, safety, welfare and environment, with due regard to legal requirements.
  (addressed in EN 45001 5.4.2; ISO Guide 25 5.2; ISO 9001 4.1.1)

- The laboratory should use materials and reagents that, where possible, should be safe for personnel and the environment.

- If the use of hazardous materials (toxic, mutagenic, radioactive) or procedures is unavoidable, appropriate measures should be taken to protect personnel and environment.

2.3 QUALITY STRATEGY OF THE LABORATORY
- The quality system of the laboratory should be described in a quality manual.
  (addressed in EN 45001 5.4.2; ISO Guide 25 5.1; ISO 9001 4.2)

- There should be a list of specific quality goals of the laboratory.
  (addressed in ISO 9001 4.2)

- The general structure of documents should be defined.
  The general format of procedures should include:
    1. Subject
    2. Purpose and scope
    3. Responsibility
    4. Definitions
    5. Action and methods
    6. References
    7. Documentation

- There should be a system for document control in which should be defined the reponsibilities for writing, evaluation, authorisation and distribution of quality system documents.
  (addressed in ISO 9001 4.4.1)

- Information appearing on each page of any document should include title, version number, page number of total number of pages, and document identification code.

- Only valid versions of procedures should be used, dated and signed by the responsible staff officer.

- The quality manual should be accessible for all personnel.
  (addressed in EN 45001 5.4.2; ISO Guide 25 5.2)

- Personnel should actively be involved in writing and changing of procedures and take notice of such changes.

- All procedures should be evaluated at least once a year.
  (addressed in EN 45001 5.4.2)

2.4 CONFIDENTIALITY

- Information about patients should be treated confidentially and measures in this respect should be defined.
  (addressed in EN 45001 5.4.6; ISO Guide 25 5.2)

2.5 IMPROPER INFLUENCE

- Measures taken to protect against improper influence (corruption) should be defined.
  (addressed in EN 45001 4; ISO Guide 25 4.2)

3. Organization and management

3.1 External relationship

3.2 Internal organizational structure

3.3 Budget management

3.4 Head of the laboratory

3.5 Professional staff and other staffing

3.1 EXTERNAL RELATIONSHIP

- There should be a description of the position of the laboratory within the parent organization, if applicable, illustrated by e.g. a diagram.
  (addressed in ISO Guide 25 5.2)

3.2 INTERNAL ORGANIZATIONAL STRUCTURE

- There should be a description of the organizational structure of the laboratory illustrated by a management diagram.
  (addressed in EN 45001 5.1, 5.4.2; ISO Guide 25 4.2; ISO 9001 4.1.2.1)

- There should be a list of all functions and their tasks, responsibilities and competencies.
  (addressed in EN 45001 5.1; ISO 9001 4.1.2.1)

3.3 BUDGET MANAGEMENT

- There should be a yearly report of the strategy, achievements and production figures of the laboratory.

- There should be a budgeting and debiting system specifying salaries, investments, other working-expenses.

- Responsibilities for budgets and efficiency should be clearly stated.

3.4 HEAD OF THE LABORATORY

- The head of the laboratory should be a specialist (e.g. clinical biochemist) recognized at national and/or international level, that is, registered in the EC4 Euro Register.

- The head of the laboratory should be responsible for management and scientific direction and should have his individual responsibility for clinical advice.

3.5 PROFESSIONAL STAFF AND OTHER STAFFING

- There should be appropiate numbers of recognized clinical biochemists as professional staff, registered at national and European level e.g. the EC4 Euro Register.

- The staff should have defined individual responsibility for consultation, choice of methodology and quality aspects of assays.

- There should be a quality officer (e.g. chief-technician) responsible for the maintenance of the quality system and manual, reporting directly to the head of the department.
(addressed in EN 45001 5.4.2; ISO Guide 25 4.2)

- There should be a safety advisor.

- There should be appropiate members of staff with the required training to ensure a satisfactory operation of service.
(addressed in EN 45001 5.1; ISO 9001 4.1.2.2)

- Regular staff meetings should be held to review services concerning organizational aspects. All staff of varying levels should be involved. Records should be kept and actions audited.

- Regular staff meetings should be held to review technical and research aspects. Records should be kept and actions audited.

4. Personnel

4.1. Job descriptions, duties and responsibilities

4.2. Service, leave and sickness planning

4.3. Education, training and development of staff

4.4. Staff appraisal system

4.1 JOB DESCRIPTIONS, DUTIES AND RESPONSIBILITIES

- There should be job descriptions for different grades of staff and these should be consistent with the management diagram.
(addressed in EN 45001 5.2; ISO Guide 25 4.2; ISO 9001 4.1.2.1)

- All staff should have an up-to-date copy of these job descriptions.
(addressed in EN 45001 5.2)

- The duties and responsibilities of all staff should be specified in the job descriptions.
(addressed in EN 45001 5.2; ISO Guide 25 4.2; ISO 9001 4.1.2.1)

4.2 SERVICE, LEAVE AND SICKNESS PLANNING

- There should be an adequate system of time scheduling of working hours and of leave and sickness planning.

4.3 EDUCATION, TRAINING AND DEVELOPMENT OF STAFF

- There should be a continuing education program for all staff. Records should be kept.
(addressed in EN 45001 5.2; ISO Guide 25 6.2; ISO 9001 4.1.2.2, 4.18)

- Professional staff takes part in appropiate post graduate education, symposia and congresses.

- There should be sufficient handbooks and scientific literature available.

4.4 STAFF APPRAISAL SYSTEM
- Personal records should be kept to ensure that there is evidence that each member of staff is regularly appraised, with clear statements of objectives.

5. Premises and environment

5.1 Laboratory space

5.2 Office space

5.3 Facilities for personnel

5.4 Facilities for patients

5.5 Safety facilities

5.6 Provisions for working environment

5.7 Storage facilities

5.1 LABORATORY SPACE
- There should be adequate bench space, in accordance with national legislation.
  (addressed in EN 45001 5.3.2; ISO Guide 25 7.1)

- There should be adequate space according to each specialisation of the laboratory.
  (addressed in ISO Guide 25 7.4)

- There should be adequate space to enable personnel to perform the required functions.
  (addressed in EN 45001 5.3.2)

- There should be space for equipment in accordance with the manufacturers recommendation.

- There should be adequate circulation space.

- There should be adequate space for sample reception and handling.

- There should be separate and adequate (according to legislation) areas for radioactive isotope work and high risk work.
  (addressed in ISO Guide 25 7.4)

- Access to the laboratories should be regulated.
  (addressed in EN 45001 5.3.2; ISO Guide 25 7.5)

- All areas should be tidy and properly clean.
  (addressed in EN 45001 5.3.2; ISO Guide 25 7.6)

5.2 OFFICE SPACE
- There should be separate office space for the head of the laboratory, the professional staff and for administration.

- There should be adequate space for computer equipment.

5.3 FACILITIES FOR PERSONNEL
- There should be adequate staff facilities for relaxation.

- There should be sufficient locker space.

- There should be sufficient toilet accommodation.

5.4 FACILITIES FOR PATIENTS
- There should be an adequate reception area with suitable access also for disabled.
- There should be adequate waiting space.
- There should be phlebotomy rooms which afford sufficient privacy.
- There should be rooms for collection of special samples from patients, where appropriate.
- There should be room for performance of dynamic function tests, where appropriate.
- There should be adequate toilet facilities for urine collection as well as hand-washing.

5.5 SAFETY FACILITIES
- There should be sufficient emergency exit facilities.
- There should be fire protection facilities.
- There should be protection against etching fluids and other high risk materials.
- There should be safety boxes for high risk reagents.
- There should be protection against hazards of biological materials.

5.6 PROVISIONS FOR WORKING ENVIRONMENT
- There should be adequate provisions for temperature control, power supply and lighting (including during power failure), ventilation, water and gases.
  (addressed in EN 45001 5.3.2; ISO Guide 25 7.3)

5.7 STORAGE FACILITIES
- There should be adequate and secure refrigerators and freezers, if critical connected to a registration and alarm system.
  (addressed in ISO 9001 4.15.3)
- There should be adequate storage facilities for glasware, supplies, reagents, specimens and other materials.
  (addressed in ISO 9001 4.15.3)

6. Equipment, materials and reagents

6.1 Administration of equipment

6.2 Purchasing of equipment

6.3 Calibration

6.4 Instructions for use and maintenance

6.5 Computer facilities

6.6 Administration of materials and reagents

6.7 Safety and environment

6.1 ADMINISTRATION OF EQUIPMENT
- There should be a list of the major equipment including identification, date received, manufacturer, price, maintenance service.
  (addressed in EN 45001 5.3.3; ISO Guide 25 8.4; ISO 9001 4.6.3)
- Equipment out of order should be properly indicated.
  (addressed in EN 45001 5.3.3; ISO Guide 25 8.2)

6.2 PURCHASING OF EQUIPMENT

- There should be a procedure for specification of requirements.
  (addressed in ISO 9001 4.6.3)

- There should be a procedure for validation of performance against specified requirements.
  (addressed in ISO 9001 4.6.4)

- There should be a procedure for assessment of suppliers (ISO certificate) including training, documentation and service.
  (addressed in ISO 9001 4.6.2)

- The criteria for selection of equipment should be established by the head of the laboratory.

6.3 CALIBRATION

- There should be calibration procedures for basic equipment like pipettes, balances, microscopes and centrifuges.
  (addressed in EN 45001 5.3.3; ISO Guide 25 9.1; ISO 9001 4.11)

- There should be procedures for calibration of major equipment. Where possible and feasible reference materials should be used for calibration. The traceability of the used calibration materials should be stated.
  (addressed in EN 45001 5.3.3; ISO Guide 25 9.2-3; ISO 9001 4.11)

6.4 INSTRUCTIONS FOR USE AND MAINTENANCE

- There should be procedures describing the use and operation of instruments.
  (addressed in EN 45001 5.3.3; ISO Guide 25 10.1; ISO 9001 4.11)

- There should be procedures for periodic maintenance.
  (addressed in EN 45001 5.3.3; ISO Guide 25 8.2; ISO 9001 4.11)

- There should be logbooks for all major equipment in which maintenance and trouble shooting should be recorded.
  (addressed in EN 45001 5.3.3; ISO Guide 25 8.2; ISO 9001 4.11)

6.5 COMPUTER FACILITIES

- There should be documentation of all hardware and software including operating instructions.
  (addressed in ISO Guide 25 10.7)

- Computer systems must be reliable and backup facilities guaranteed.
  (addressed in EN 45001 5.4.1; ISO Guide 25 10.7)

- Systems should be validated for required functions.
  (addressed in ISO Guide 25 10.7)

- There should be adequate facilities for the storage of software back-ups and databases.
  (addressed in ISO Guide 25 10.7)

- Access to databases should be protected for non-authorised persons.
  (addressed in ISO Guide 25 10.7)

- There should be defined access to different authorisation levels.

6.6 ADMINISTRATION OF MATERIALS AND REAGENTS

- There should be procedures for selecting reagents and materials.
  (addressed in ISO 9001 4.6.1)

- There should be procedures for purchasing and ordering of reagents and materials.
  (addressed in ISO Guide 25 10.8; ISO 9001 4.6.3)

- The criteria of these should be established by the head of the laboratory.

- There should be a procedure for assessment of suppliers (ISO certificate).
  (addressed in ISO 9001 4.6.2)

- There should be procedures to ensure that reagents and materials are checked for condition upon delivery, that they are stored correctly (temperature and other conditions) and that they are used only within the expiry date.
  (addressed in ISO 9001 4.6.4)

- There should be procedures to control inventory (minimum/maximum stock).

- Reagents and materials should be correctly identified and dated including name of responsible organization or person, name, concentration, date of first use, date of expiry, danger/safety indication.
  (addressed in ISO 9001 4.6.3)

6.7 SAFETY AND ENVIRONMENT

- There should be appropriate danger indications on all reagents and materials if toxic, radioactive, carcinogenic or mutagenic.

- There should be procedures for separate collection of different types of waste including reagents, wash-waste, needles and infectious materials, and this should be administrated.
  (addressed in ISO Guide 25 11.4)

7. Pre-analytical phase

7.1 User information

7.2 Consultation and efficacy

7.3 Repertoire

7.4 Request procedures

7.5 Information and preparation of patients

7.6 Sample collection

7.7 Sample transport and handling

7.8 Experimental testing

7.9 Confidentiality and safety

7.1 USER INFORMATION

- There should be a user information system (e.g. handbook) which will contain appropriate information from the succeeding paragraphs.

7.2 CONSULTATION AND EFFICACY

- Consultation concerning efficacy of tests, repeat frequency and required type of sample should be available at all times.

- There should be regular meetings of professional staff with the clinical staff regarding the use of the laboratory and consultation on scientific matters.

- The professional staff should participate in clinical rounds for consultation on efficacy in individual cases as well as in general.

- The consultation function should be part of medical audit.

7.3 REPERTOIRE

- There should be a list of the stat and 24 hours repertoire.

- There should be a list of the repertoire of all available tests, including required specimen and sample volume, special precautions, normal turn-around time, reference ranges.
- There should be a defined role for the laboratory in the validation, assessment and quality control of point of care testing.
- The repertoires should be adjusted regularly and be part of medical audit.

7.4 REQUEST PROCEDURES
- There should be procedures for urgent and routine requests.
- The request form should be designed in order to obtain necessary information for identification of the patient, the requesting physician, requested tests and clinical information.
- The request form should facilitate efficacy by its lay-out (e.g. disease oriented).
- In the request form specific required conditions for the patient for individual tests (e.g. fasting) should be indicated.

7.5 INFORMATION AND PREPARATION OF PATIENTS
- There should be information available for patients if specific diets or other preparation is required.
- There should be information available for patients concerning collection of urine, faeces, semen.
- There should be information for patients concerning opening hours and location of the laboratory.
- Waiting time for the patients should meet defined criteria.

7.6 SAMPLE COLLECTION
- There should be a procedure describing all aspects of blood and other specimen collection including patient identification, patient position, sampling technique, and biological safety aspects.
- There should be a procedure for unique identification of samples and subdivided samples including labelling and date and time registration of sample and requests.
  (addressed in EN 45001 5.4.5; ISO Guide 25 11.1)
- There should be a list containing for each test information about the type of specimen, the type of tube and anticoagulant, collecting temperature, and the amount of sample needed.
  (addressed in EN 45001 5.4.5; ISO Guide 25 10.5)

7.7 SAMPLE TRANSPORT AND HANDLING
- There should be procedures for transport and handling of samples including required temperature, protection from light, stoppering precautions, allowable time lag before pre-treatment (e.g. centrifugation, deproteinisation) or assay and storage conditions.
  (addressed in EN 45001 5.4.5; ISO Guide 25 11.3)
- There should be procedures to minimize the risk of interchange of samples and subdivided samples.
  (addressed in EN 45001 5.4.5; ISO Guide 25 11.3)
- There should be procedures for sending samples to other laboratories, including required pre-treatment and precautions, urgency of transport, required forms and arrangements.
  (addressed in EN 45001 5.4.7; ISO Guide 25 14.1)
- If a sample is assayed elsewhere, enough information should be given and the mutual responsibilities should be defined.
  (addressed in EN 45001 5.4.7; ISO Guide 25 14.2)

7.8 Experimental testing
- There should be procedures for experimental testing, including regulation for informed consent and involvement of the medical ethical committee.

- Testing should be performed adhering to strict protocols.

- If different conditions with respect to routine laboratory procedures exist, they should be made explicit.

7.9 Confidentiality and safety
- Regulations to guarantee biological safety of patients, phlebotomists and technicians should be present, known and audited.

- Confidentiality of patients should be guaranteed.
  (addressed in EN 45001 5.4.6; ISO Guide 25 5.2)

- All accidents with respect to sampling, transportation and handling of samples should be documented.
  (addressed in EN 45001 5.4.5; ISO Guide 25 11.2)

8. Analytical phase

8.1 Validation

8.2 Calibration and traceability of methods

8.3 Working procedures

8.4 Quality control and assessment

8.5 Authorisation

8.6 Archiving

8.7 Disposal of samples

8.1 Validation
- On introduction of a new analytical procedure the performance should be validated against specified requirements.
  (addressed in EN 45001 5.4.1; ISO Guide 25 10.2; ISO 9001 4.9.1)

- Such validation should include, where possible, determination of systematic bias against reference materials or otherwise stated values, limit of detection, limits of determination, within- and between-run reproducibility, interfering substances, robustness.
  (addressed in ISO Guide 25 10.2)

- Limitations of applicability for different materials should be stated.
  (addressed in ISO Guide 25 10.1)

- Equipment should be validated by the manufacturer with respect to basic functions such as temperature control, wavelength characteristics and pipetting performance. The validation summary should be available upon request.
  (addressed in EN 45001 5.3.3; ISO Guide 25 9.1)

8.2 Calibration and traceability of methods
- Calibration frequency and calibration method should be stated e.g. in the working procedure.
  (addressed in EN 45001 5.3.3; ISO Guide 25 9.1; ISO 9001 11)

- Calibration materials and their traceability should be stated.
  (addressed in EN 45001 5.3.3; ISO Guide 25 9.2; ISO 9001 11)

- Origin of absorption coefficients, factors and their traceability should be documented.
  (addressed in EN 45001 5.3.3; ISO Guide 25 9.2)

8.3 WORKING PROCEDURES

- Working procedures should be available for all assays.
  (addressed in EN 45001 5.4.1; ISO Guide 25 10.1; ISO 9001 9.1)

- Working procedures should be available at the bench.
  (addressed in EN 45001 5.4.1; ISO Guide 25 10.1)

- There should be working procedures for logistic procedures, analytical procedures including measurement and observation techniques, and instrument procedures.
  (addressed in EN 45001 5.4.1; ISO Guide 25 10.1; ISO 9001 9.1)

- Working procedures should comprise, if applicable:
  0. Title
  1. Subject
  2. Purpose and scope
  3. Responsibilities
  4. Definitions
  5. Action and methods
     - 5.1 Clinical relevance
     - 5.2 Reaction principle
     - 5.3 Safety and environment aspects
     - 5.4 Reagents, calibrants and control materials
     - 5.5 Equipment and means
     - 5.6 Sample taking, specimen requirements, identification
     - 5.7 Instructions including start-up, precautions, pretreatment, analysis, detection limit, lower and higher limit, disposal of waste, remarks and error codes, trouble shooting
     - 5.8 Results, units, registration, calculations, particularities
     - 5.9 Reporting, report values, emergency limits, reference limits
     - 5.10 Quality control and assessment: intra-laboratory control (materials, acceptance limits), external quality assessment
     - 5.11 Validation: referral to documents stating within run and between run variation, accuracy, detection limit, linearity, interfering substances
     - 5.12 Remarks
  6. References
  7. Documentation

8.4 QUALITY CONTROL AND ASSESSMENT

- There should be a system of internal quality control.
  (addressed in EN 45001 5.4.2; ISO Guide 25 5.6; ISO 9001 10.2)

- Criteria against which analytical processes (measurement and also observation) are judged should be stated for example in the working procedures.

- Such criteria should preferably be based on biological variance.

- Internal quality control results should be checked and kept at the bench according to the working procedures.
  (addressed in ISO Guide 25 5.6; ISO 9001 10.2)

- The laboratory should take part in valid external quality assessment schemes (EQAS), preferably those organized by the profession, and covering the repertoire.
  (addressed in EN 45001 5.4.2; ISO Guide 25 5.6)

- Internal quality control results, also from point of care equipment, and EQAS results should be regularly evaluated in technical staff meetings and actions taken should be documented.
  (addressed in ISO Guide 25 5.6)

8.5 AUTHORISATION
- Measurements and observations should be verified by competent technical staff, taking into account internal quality control results, instrument flags, linearity, limits of determination.

- First authorisation should be done by senior staff.

- Professional staff should authorize final reports.
  (addressed in EN 45001 5.4.3; ISO Guide 25 13.2)

8.6 ARCHIVING
- Outdated procedures should be archived for at least two years.

- Request forms should be archived for at least three months.

- Worklists containing intermediate results and observations should be archived for at least three months.
  (addressed in EN 45001 5.4.4; ISO Guide 25 12.1; ISO 9001 4.16)

- Results should be archived for a period of twice the medically informative period, with a minimum of one year and an advised maximum of ten years.

- Archives should be organized to ensure patient confidentiality.
  (addressed in EN 45001 5.4.4; ISO Guide 25 12.2)

- Internal quality control results should be archived for at least one year.

- External quality assessment results should be archived for at least five years.

- Destruction of archives should ensure confidentiality.

8.7 DISPOSAL OF SAMPLES
- Patient material should be considered and treated as potentially infectious.

- Specimens, needles and blood contaminated disposables should be disposed in special containers and be treated as infectious waste.
  (addressed in EN 45001 5.4.5; ISO Guide 25 11.4)

9. Post-analytical phase

9.1 Reporting procedures

9.2 Correction procedures

9.3 Turn-around time

9.4 Reference values

9.5 Interpretation and consultation

9.6 Archiving

9.7 Confidentiality

9.1 REPORTING PROCEDURES
- There should be procedures for reporting of results.

- Report items should include:
  Laboratory name
  Patient name and address
  Requesting person
  Test description
  Sample kind
  Sampling date and time
  Result(s)
  Interpretational comments if necessary
  Signature of professional
  (addressed in EN 45001 5.4.3; ISO Guide 25 13.2)

- Reporting of results should be definitive only after the complete analytical authorization procedure, including authorization by professional staff.
  (addressed in EN 45001 5.4.3; ISO Guide 25 13.2)

- Stat results, results obtained in out of hours service and results outside alarm limits should be reported as soon as possible, but only after verification by a competent technician.

- Reporting of results by telephone should be limited and followed by written, printed or electronic reporting as soon as possible.

9.2 CORRECTION PROCEDURES

- Reported results should only be corrected by authorized professionals.
  (addressed in EN 45001 5.4.3; ISO Guide 25 13.5)

- Correction of the results should be reported as soon as possible to the requesting physician.
  (addressed in ISO Guide 25 13.6)

- Corrected results should be clearly indicated as such in the report.
  (addressed in EN 45001 5.4.3; ISO Guide 25 13.5)

- In case of a wrong result there should always be a procedure to investigate the underlying cause.
  (addressed in ISO 9001 4.14)

9.3 TURN-AROUND TIME

- The requesting physician should be familiar with the normal reporting time for assays.

- Turn-around times for stat and routine tests should be audited regularly.

- The turn-around time for assays sent to other laboratories should be known and checked.

- Turn-around times should be part of medical audit.

9.4 REFERENCE VALUES

- Reference values should be available for all assays, where relevant.

- The reference values should be checked by the laboratory.

9.5 INTERPRETATION AND CONSULTATION

- Consultation concerning interpretation of results and advice on further investigation should be available at all times.

- There should be regular meetings of professional staff with the clinical staff regarding use of the laboratory and interpretation of results.

- The professional staff should participate in clinical rounds for consultation concerning interpretation in individual cases.

- Professional staff should participate in medical and clinical audit.

- Professional staff should add interpretational remarks to reported results if necessary, e.g. warnings should be added to the report when pathological pitfalls or interfering substances are suspected.

9.6 ARCHIVING

- Results should be archived for a period of twice the medically informative period, with a minimum of one year and an advised maximum of ten years.
  (addressed in EN 45001 5.4.4; ISO Guide 25 12.1)

- Archives should be organized to ensure patient confidentiality.
  (addressed in EN 45001 5.4.6; ISO Guide 25 12.2)

- There should be adequate back up procedures for electronic archives.

- The archive should be protected against damage.
  (addressed in EN 45001 5.4.4; ISO Guide 25 12.2)

9.7 CONFIDENTIALITY

- There should be a procedure regarding confidentiality of results.
  (addressed in EN 45001 5.4.6; ISO Guide 25 12.2)

10. Evaluation of the quality system

10.1 Internal audit

10.2 Internal and external complaints

10.3 External audit

10.1 INTERNAL AUDIT

- There should be a system of planned internal audits.
  (addressed in EN 45001 5.4.2; ISO Guide 25 5.3; ISO 9001 4.17)

- Results of internal audits should be documented and responsible staff should be informed.
  (addressed in ISO 9001 4.17)

- There should be documented activities in concordance with the results of internal audits.
  (addressed in EN 45001 5.4.2; ISO Guide 25 5.3; ISO 9001 4.17)

- There should be procedures for corrective actions and assessment of their effectiveness.

- All procedures should be checked at least once a year.
  (addressed in ISO Guide 25 5.4)

- There should be a checklist of all items and aims described in the handbook and this should be checked once a year.

10.2 INTERNAL AND EXTERNAL COMPLAINTS

- There should be a low threshold system for reporting internal (from within the laboratory) (near) accidents, complaints and ideas.

- Internal (near) accidents, complaints and ideas should be registered.
  (addressed in ISO Guide 25 16.1)

- External (from outside the laboratory) accidents, near accidents and complaints should be registered.
  (addressed in ISO Guide 25 16.1)

- Internal and external complaints and ideas should be discussed in staff meetings and actions taken documented.
  (addressed in EN 45001 5.4.2; ISO Guide 25 16.1)

- Professional staff should decide whether reported (near) accidents should lead to immediate measures concerning organization or consultation.

10.3 EXTERNAL AUDIT

- Professional staff should take part in medical audit.

- The laboratory should strive after inspection and accreditation according to EC4 approved criteria.
  (addressed in EN 45001 6.2)

- Professional staff should be prepared to function as auditor(s) in the external accreditation system on the basis claim of expenses.

Index